STEP BY STEP
TRANSITION GUIDE

Journal & Workbook

800.578-5939
www.AlkalineLifestyle.com

Table of Contents

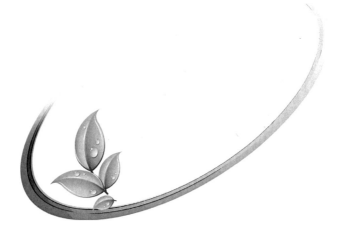

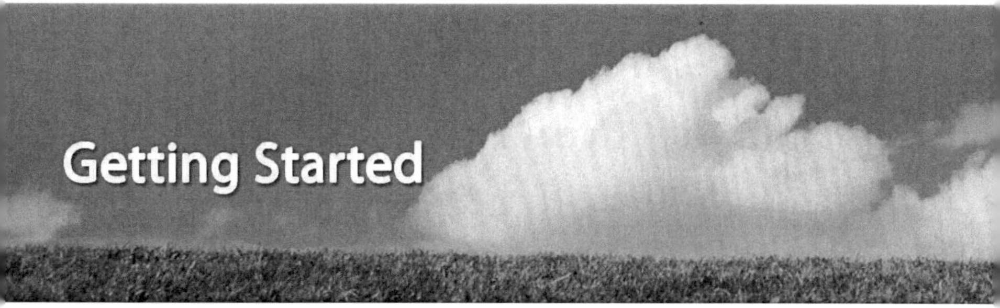

Getting Started

Goal setting provides a focus for your transition to the Alkaline Lifestyle. Take a moment now to think through your goals.

Choose a big goal to reach for – make it attainable, yet big enough so that you will celebrate your accomplishments when you reach it.

Examples of big goals include:

- Lose 20 pounds
- Run a mile without stopping
- Attain an overall alkaline state
- Wake up feeling happy

Write your big goal ideas below:

_____

_____

_____

_____

_____

_____

_____

Now transform your big goal into a statement of intention. Pick the goal that appeals to you the most. Write it in the statement, below.

I am committed to _____

_____

_____

(and write in your big goal)

Now think about your reasons for choosing this goal. Why is this goal important to you? Reflect and write down your thoughts below.

_____

_____

_____

_____

_____

_____

Now think about how you will feel when you attain this goal. What emotions come to mind? Take an imaginary trip and imagine how it will feel to run a mile without losing your breath, how it will feel to be able to play with your children without getting winded or how it will feel to be at your goal weight.

What steps do you think you will need to take to achieve this goal? Write them down below. For example, to lose 10 pounds, you will need to focus on healthy alkaline eating. To run a mile without losing your breath you will need to begin an exercise program. Other steps may be to contact one of the professionals on the Alkaline Lifestyle website and seek information; read and complete the steps and exercises in this workbook; purchase alkaline foods and supplements; and more.

1. _____

2. _____

3. _____

4. _____

5. _____

6. _____

7. _____

8. _____

9. _____

10. _____

What will you do to celebrate your success once you achieve your goal?

1. _____

_____

2. _____

_____

3. _____

_____

Write out your goal on this page. Print it out and hang it where you can see it every day!

I, _____am committed
to achieving my goal of _____

_____

_____

Each day, I will _____

_____,

_____, and _____

_____

_____

to achieve my goal.

When I have achieved my goal, I will celebrate by

_____

_____

_____

I have the power to choose daily actions that lead to success. With every day, I am closer to my goal!

My Starting Point

List your information here. We'll check this information each week, and you can record progress in your journal.

Today's date:_____

My height:_____

My current weight:_____

My BMI:_____

My pH today:_____

The optimal range is 6.8 to 7.2._____

BMI CHART

Weight in Pounds

Height	120	130	140	150	160	170	180	190	200	210	220	230	240	250
4'6"	29	31	34	36	39	41	43	46	48	51	53	56	58	60
4'8"	27	29	31	34	36	38	40	43	45	47	49	52	54	56
4'10"	25	27	29	31	34	36	38	40	42	44	46	48	50	52
5'0"	23	25	27	29	31	33	35	37	39	41	43	45	47	49
5'2"	22	24	26	27	29	31	33	35	37	38	40	42	44	46
5'4"	21	22	24	26	28	29	31	33	34	36	38	40	41	43
5'6"	19	21	23	24	26	27	29	31	32	34	36	37	39	40
5'8"	18	20	21	23	24	26	27	29	30	32	34	35	37	38
5'10"	17	19	20	22	23	24	26	27	29	30	32	33	35	36
6'0"	16	18	19	20	22	23	24	26	27	28	30	31	33	34
6'2"	15	17	18	19	21	22	23	24	26	27	28	30	31	32
6'4"	15	16	17	18	20	21	22	23	24	26	27	28	29	30
6'6"	14	15	16	17	19	20	21	22	23	24	25	27	28	29
6'8"	13	14	15	17	18	19	20	21	22	23	24	25	26	28

Height in Feet and Inches

- Underweight
- Healthy Weight
- Overweight
- Obese

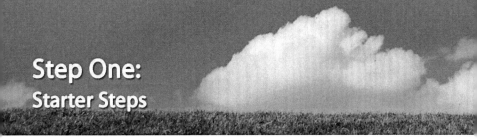

Step One:
Starter Steps

Step 1 consists of several 'starter steps' to get you started on the Alkaline Lifestyle.

The first exercise is determine your current pH status and record it on the **My Starting Point** page (page 12)

How do you feel about your starting point?

_____

_____

_____

_____

_____

_____

_____

_____

_____

Record Your Food

One way to pinpoint the most acidic foods you are currently eating – and the first you should eliminate from your diet – is to log your daily food intake. Use this page to record your food for at least one day but preferable over three or more days. Make as many copies of these pages as you need.

Breakfast:_____
_____
_____

Lunch:_____
_____
_____

Dinner:_____
_____
_____

Snacks:_____

_____

_____

Beverages:_____

_____

_____

Any special events happening today that might affect
my food choices such as a party, dinner out with friends,
or business lunch? _____

_____

_____

How much water did I drink? What type of water did I
drink? _____

_____

Do I drink coffee, tea, alcohol or soft drinks? How much?

_____

_____

Choosing Alkaline Foods

Compare your daily food intake to the **Acid and Alkaline Food Chart** on pages 20 & 21.

(Chart prepared by Dr. Russell Jaffe, Fellow, Health Studies Collegium.)

Grab two different colored pens or pencils. Put a check mark in one color to indicate foods on your daily intake that are ACID and a check mark in a different color next to foods that are ALKALINE.

Add up all the check marks:_____

Add up the ACID colored checkmarks:_____

Subtract the ACID marks from the total. This is your ALKALINE INTAKE. _____

Ideally, 80% of your daily foods should be ALKALINE and the remaining 20% may be Acidic.

How does your typical day stack up now?

_____

_____

_____

_____

_____

What changes can you make to push the balance more towards alkaline?

_____

_____

_____

_____

_____

Alkaline & Acid Food Chart

Food Category	Most Alkaline	More Alkaline	Low Alkaline	Lowest Alkaline
Spice/Herb	Baking Soda	Spices/Cinnamon Valerian Licorice •Black Cohash Agave	•Herbs (most):Arnica, Bergamot, Echinacea Chrysanthemum, Ephedra, Feverfew, Goldenseal, Lemon-grass, Aloe Vera, Nettle, Angelica	White Willow Bard Slippery Elm Artemisia Annua
Preservative Beverage Sweetner Vinegar	Sea Salt Mineral Water	•Kambucha Molasses Soy Sauce	•Green or **Mu** Tea Rice Syrup Apple Cider Vinegar	Sulfite Ginger Tea •Sucanat •Umeboshi Vinegar
Therapeutic	•Umeboshi Plum		•Sake	•Algae, Blue Green
Processed Dairy Cow/Human Soy Goat/Sheep				•Ghee (Clarified Butter) Human Breast Milk
Egg			•Quail Egg	•Duck Egg
Meat Game Fish/Shell Fish				
Fowl				
Grain Cereal Grass				Oat "Grain Coffee" •Quinoa, Wild Rice, •Amaranth, Japonica Rice
Nut Seed/Sprout Oil	Pumpkin Seed	Poppy Seed, Cashew, Chestnut, Pepper	Primrose Oil, Sesame Seed, Cod Liver Oil, Almond, •Sprout	Avocado Oil, Seeds (most), Coconut Oil, Olive/Macadamia Oil, Linseed/Flax Oil
Bean Vegetable Legume Pulse Root	Lentil, Brocoflower, •Seaweed, Onion/ Miso, •Daikon/ Taro Root, Sea Vegetables (other) Dandelion Greens, •Burdock/•Lotus Root, Sweet Potato/Yam	Kohirabi, Parsnip/Taro, Garlic, Asparagus, Kale/Parsley, Endive/Arugula, Mustard Greens, Jerusalem Artichoke, Ginger Root, Broccoli	Potato/Bell Pepper, Mushroom/Fungi, Cauliflower, Cabbage, Rutabaga, •Salsify/Ginseng, Eggplant, Pumpkin, Collard Greens	Brussel Sprout, Beet, Chive/Cilantro, Celery/Scalion, Okra/Cucumber, Turnip Greens, Squash, Artichoke, Lettuce, Jicama
Citrus Fruit Fruit	Lime, Nectarine, Persimmon, Rasp-berry, Watermelon, Tangerine, Pineapple	Grapefruit, Cante-loupe, Honeydew, Cit-rus, Olive, •Dewberry, Loganberry, Mango	Lemon, Pear, Avocado, Apple, Blackberry, Cherry, Peach, Papaya, Acai Berry, Goji Berry	Orange, Apricot, Banana, Blueberry, Pineapple Juice, Raisin, Currant, Grape, Strawberry

•Therapeutic, gourmet, or exotic items

Alkaline & Acid Food Chart

Food Category	Lowest Acid	Low Acid	More Acid	Most Acid
Spice/Herb	Curry	Vanilla, Stevia	Nutmeg	Pudding/Jam/Jelly
Preservative Beverage Sweetner Vinegar	*MSG* Kona Coffee Honey/Maple Syrup Rice Vinegar	*Benzoate* *Alcohol*, Black Tea Balsamic Vinegar	*Aspartame* *Coffee* *Saccharin* Red Wine Vinegar	*Table Salt (NaCL)* *Beer, 'Soda'* Yeast/Hops/Malt Sugar/Cocoa *White/Acetic Vinegar*
Therapeutic		Antihistamines	Psychotropics	Antibiotics
Processed Dairy Cow/Human Soy Goat/Sheep	Cream/Butter Yogurt Goat/Sheep Cheese	Cow Milk Aged Cheese Soy Cheese Goat Milk	•Casein, Milk Protein, Cottage Cheese Soy Milk	Processed Cheese Ice Cream
Egg	Chicken Egg			
Meat Game Fish/Shell Fish	Gelatin/Organs •Venison Fish	Lamb/Mutton Boar/Elk/•Game Meat Mullusks Shell Fish (Whole)	Pork/Veal Bear •Mussel/ Squid	Beef Shell Fish (Processed) •Lobster
Fowl	Wild Duck	Goose/Turkey	Chicken	Pheasant
Grain Cereal Grass	•Triticale, Millet, Kasha, Brown Rice	Buckwheat, Wheat, Spelt/Teff/Kamut Farina/Semolina White Rice	Maize, Barley Groat Corn Rye Oat Bran	Barley Processed Flour
Nut Seed/Sprout Oil	Pumpkin Seed Oil Grape Seed Oil Sunflower Oil, Pine Nut, Canola Oil	Almond Oil, Sesame Oil, Safflower Oil, Tapioca, •Seitan or Tofu	Pistachio Seed Chestnut Oil, *Lard*, Pecan, Palm Kernel Oil	Cottonseed Oil/Meal Hazelnut, Walnut, Brazil Nut *Fried Food*
Bean Vegetable Legume Pulse Root	Spinach, Fava Bean, Kidney Bean, Black-eyed Pea, String/Wax Beach, Zucchini, Chutney, Rhubarb	Split Pea, Pinto Bean, White Bean, Navy/ Red Bean, Aduki Bean, Lima or Mung Bean, Chard	Green Pea, Peanut, Snow Pea, Legumes (other), Car- rot, ChickPea/ Garbanzo	Soybean Carob
Citrus Fruit Fruit	Coconut, Guava, Pickled Fruit, Dry Fruit, Fig, Persimmon Juice, Cherimoya, Date	Plum Prune Tomato	Cranberry Pomegranate	

21

Italicized items are NOT recommended

The 80/20 Fill Your Plate Graph

Ideally, your food intake should be at least 80% alkaline and 20% acidic.

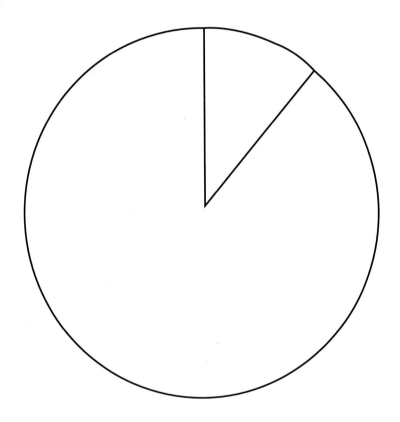

On the plate graphic on your left, write the names of foods in the 80% area from the ALKALINE section of the food chart that appeal to you. Write as many as you can fit.

In the 20% section, choose a handful of foods that you feel you just can't give up right now.

Use this as your guideline to choosing menus, recipes and more.

Reflections

What did you learn this week on the Alkaline Lifestyle?

_____

_____

_____

_____

How are you feeling about your healthy transformation?

_____

_____

_____

What changes are you making this week?

_____

_____

_____

Do you have any questions? Write them below, then go to **www.alkalinelifestyle.com** and ask the experts.

_____

_____

_____

Action Steps

Suggested Step 1 Action Steps
1. Complete the food log for at least 1 but preferably several days.
2. Identify current Acid and Alkaline Foods.
3. Create a list of enticing Alkaline foods from the food list
4. Begin weaning yourself off of coffee, tea, alcohol, sugar, artificial sweeteners (if necessary).
5. Write down your questions.
6. Ask the nutrition and fitness experts on our website your questions.

This week, I will:

1. _____

2. _____

3. _____

4. _____

5. _____

6. _____

7. _____

8. _____

9. _____

10. _____

Weekly Check In

Today's date:_____

My height:_____

My current weight:_____

My BMI:_____

My pH today:_____

The optimal range is 6.8 to 7.2._____

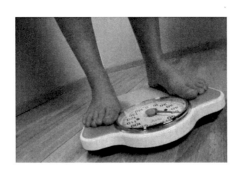

Step Two:
Fuel to Start Your Day: Breakfast

Please read Step 2 in the Step by Step book before completing these exercises.

What do you normally eat for breakfast?

_____

_____

How do you feel afterwards?

_____

_____

_____

_____

Why is it important for you to eat in accordance with nature's phases?

_____

_____

_____

_____ 27

Here's your plate at breakfast. Using the Acid and Alkaline Food chart, write in potential breakfast foods that are Alkaline on the 80% portion of the circle. You can fill your whole plate with Alkaline foods if you wish.

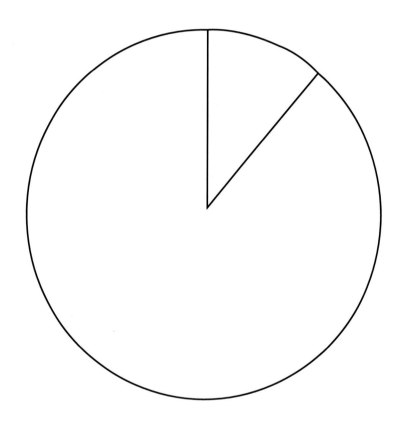

Review the Menu sent to you each week and the Recipes in the accompanying book and online.

List 7 Breakfast Recipes here that appeal to you. Make sure you note where to find them!

1. _____

2. _____

3. _____

4. _____

5. _____

6. _____

7. _____

Now PRINT THEM OUT and staple them together to form one week of Breakfast Choices.

That's your personal Breakfast Book for the Alkaline Lifestyle!

Reflections

What did you learn this week on the Alkaline Lifestyle?

_____

_____

_____

_____

How are you feeling about your healthy transformation?

_____

_____

_____

_____

What changes are you making this week?

_____

_____

_____

Do you have any questions? Write them below, then go to **www.alkalinelifestyle.com** and ask the experts.

_____

_____

_____

Action Steps

This week, I will take the following action steps to incorporate the Alkaline Lifestyle information into my daily routine:

1._____

2._____

3._____

4._____

5._____

6._____

7._____

8._____

Weekly Check In

Today's date:_____

My height:_____

My current weight:_____

My BMI:_____

My pH today:_____

The optimal range is 6.8 to 7.2._____

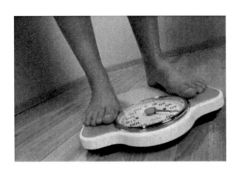

Step Three:
Alkalizing on the Go: Lunch

Look back at your food log in Step 1.

List your typical lunches on work days:

_____

_____

_____

_____

_____

List your typical lunches on week days:

_____

_____

_____

_____

Compare these to the Acid and Alkaline food chart. How
do they stack up? Are they acidic overall, or alkaline?

_____

_____

_____

What challenges do you face as you choose Alkaline lunches? Some common challenges are difficulty finding healthy alkaline foods, pressure from friends/coworkers/family to eat what they're eating, etc.

_____

_____

_____

_____

What can you say if pressed to eat off your plan?

_____

_____

_____

What action steps can you take to ensure you have alkaline food choices at lunch?

_____

_____

_____

_____

_____

Using the Acid and Alkaline Food chart, write in potential lunch foods that are Alkaline on the 80% portion of the circle. You can fill your whole plate with Alkaline foods if you wish.

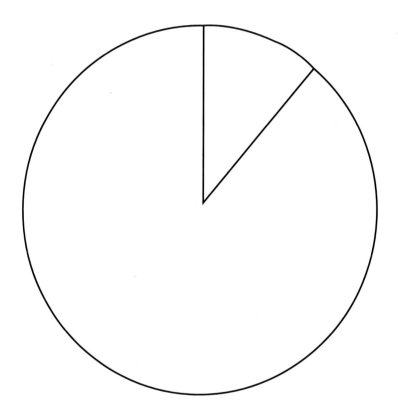

Review the Menu sent to you each week and the Recipes in the accompanying book and online.

List 7 Lunch Recipes here that appeal to you. Make sure you note where to find them!

1. _____

2. _____

3. _____

4. _____

5. _____

6. _____

7. _____

Now review your Lunch choices. Which ones are best for alkalizing on the go? Can you carry these to work?

List 3 below.

1. _____

2. _____

3. _____

Now PRINT each recipe and staple them together. You should have a booklet with 10 possible ALKALINE Lunch Choices. This is your personal guide.

Reflections

What did you learn this week on the Alkaline Lifestyle?

_____

_____

_____

_____

How are you feeling about your healthy transformation?

_____

_____

_____

_____

What changes are you making this week?

_____

_____

_____

Do you have any questions? Write them below, then go to **www.alkalinelifestyle.com** and ask the experts.

_____

_____

_____

Action Steps

This week, I will take the following action steps to incorporate the Alkaline Lifestyle information into my daily routine:

1._____

2._____

3._____

4._____

5._____

6._____

7._____

8._____

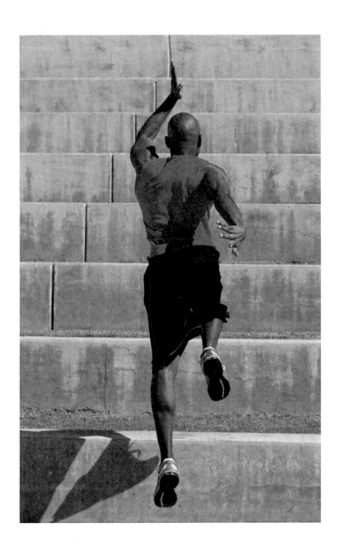

Weekly Check In

Today's date:_____

My height:_____

My current weight:_____

My BMI:_____

My pH today:_____

The optimal range is 6.8 to 7.2._____

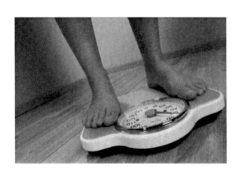

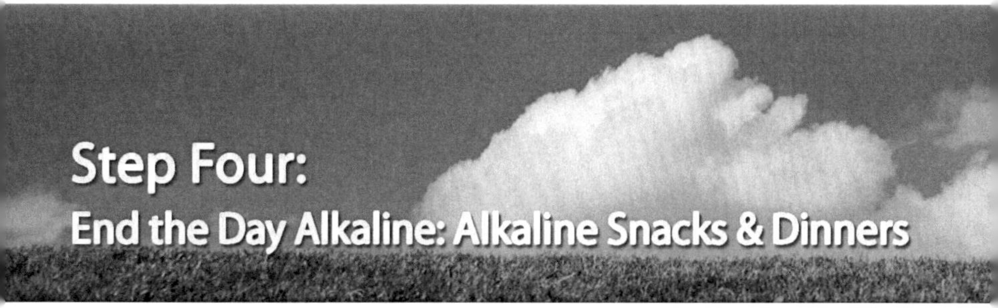

Step Four:
End the Day Alkaline: Alkaline Snacks & Dinners

Dinner may be the trickiest meal of the day to eat alkaline if you are preparing meals for the entire family. You may need to transition the family gradually into an alkaline meal plan.

Single people may skip this section and go to the pages on choosing and recording Dinner selections. The term "family" is used here to denote all people living in the household – partners, spouses, children and anyone who joins together to form your household.

Do you sit down together as a family to share a meal?

_____

_____

_____

What are typical family dinners like at your home?

_____

_____

_____

_____

Do you have at least a half hour of time to prepare a meal?

_____

_____

If not – why not?

_____

_____

_____

_____

Can you adjust your schedule at all or ask for help with meal preparations or other tasks to make time to prepare a meal?

_____

_____

_____

_____

What foods do the other people in your home love? Are these foods that you can include in dinner, keeping in mind that the average of your meals for the day should be 80% alkaline and 20% acidic?

_____

_____

_____

_____

_____

If you have young children in your home, as you look at the Acid-Alkaline Food Chart, what Alkaline Foods on the chart do your children eat now?

_____

_____

_____

_____

_____

If none, can you begin introducing a few to them each week without making a big fuss over it? Can you make it fun, an adventure?

_____

_____

If your spouse or partner doesn't want to participate in the Alkaline Lifestyle, can you set aside a shelf for "their" food and mentally make it "off limits?"

_____

_____

_____

If you try this – does it set you up for craving the food or are you okay with it?

_____

_____

_____

If you end up craving the food, what strategies can you take to shake off the cravings?

_____

_____

_____

_____

_____

Snack Strategy

It's important to keep your body fueled throughout the day. Snacks can be a healthy lifestyle choice if you select alkaline-based snacks and keep portion sizes reasonable.

Look at the Acid-Alkaline Food Chart. List 10 alkaline-rich snacks on the next page:

Some ideas of alkaline-rich snacks include:

- Green smoothies
- Kale chips
- Pumpkin seeds, roasted, toasted or spicy
- Vegetable sticks and dip
- Grapefruit slices
- Raw almonds

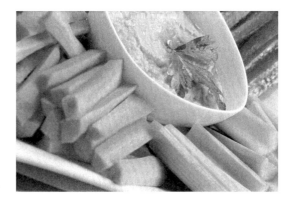

1._____

2._____

3._____

4._____

5._____

6._____

7._____

8._____

9._____

10._____

Which ones are portable?

_____

_____

_____

_____

_____

Review the Recipes online and in the book and find a few snack ideas.

Using the Acid and Alkaline Food chart, write in potential dinner meals that are Alkaline on the 80% portion of the circle. You can fill your whole plate with Alkaline foods if you wish.

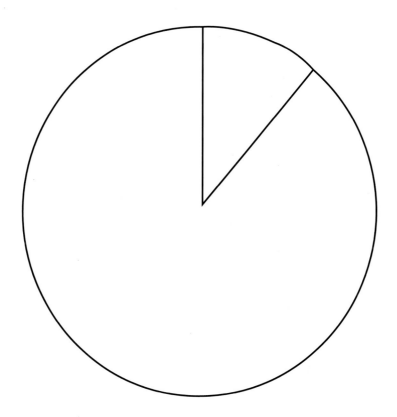

Review the Menu sent to you each week and the Recipes in the accompanying book and online.

List 7 Dinner Recipes here that appeal to you. Make sure you note where to find them!

1. _____

2. _____

3. _____

4. _____

5. _____

6. _____

7. _____

Now review your Dinner choices. Which ones are best for alkalizing on the go? Can you carry these to work?

List 3 below.

1. _____

2. _____

3. _____

Now PRINT each recipe and staple them together. You should have a booklet with 10 possible ALKALINE Dinner Choices. This is your personal guide.

Print your Snack recipes and ideas too.

Reflections

What did you learn this week on the Alkaline Lifestyle?

_____

_____

_____

_____

How are you feeling about your healthy transformation?

_____

_____

_____

What changes are you making this week?

_____

_____

_____

Do you have any questions? Write them below, then go to **www.alkalinelifestyle.com** and ask the experts.

_____

_____

_____

Action Steps

This week, I will take the following action steps to incorporate the Alkaline Lifestyle information into my daily routine:

1._____

2._____

3._____

4._____

5._____

6._____

7._____

8._____

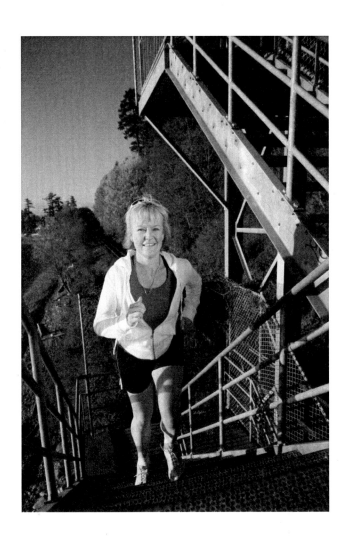

Weekly Check In

Today's date:_____

My height:_____

My current weight:_____

My BMI:_____

My pH today:_____

The optimal range is 6.8 to 7.2._____

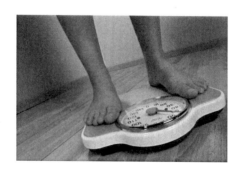

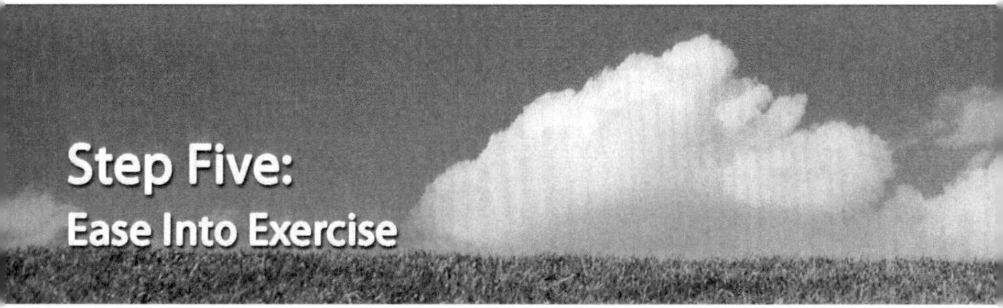

Step Five:
Ease Into Exercise

In Step 5, you will incorporate healthy aerobic activity into your lifestyle. Be sure to check with your health care provider if you have any disabilities, diseases or medical conditions. He or she will advise you on the best way to incorporate exercise into your life.

The Alkaline Lifestyle website also provides access to a certified fitness trainer who will help you develop a fitness program that fits your lifestyle and current fitness level. Do use all of the resources available to you. We care about your success!

Do you exercise now?

_____

Why or why not?

_____

_____

_____

What is stopping you from exercising more?

_____

_____

_____ 53

What can you do to fit exercise into your day?

_____

_____

_____

On a scale of 1 to 10, with 1 being "I do not like this at all" and 10 being "I love it!", assign a number to each of the following:

- Structured exercise activities, such as lessons or classes? _____

- Time spent outdoors to exercise, such as walking, hiking, etc? _____

- Competition – games, sports, team sports? _____

- The social atmosphere of a gym? _____

See any high numbers or 10's anywhere? Focus on areas you like.

List any exercises you can think of that fit any of the statements for which you assigned a 5 or higher:

_____

_____

_____

_____

_____

What do you need to start any of these? Do you need equipment, special clothing, a gym membership?

_____

_____

_____

_____

What steps can you take to obtain whatever it is you need to do the exercise you've selected?

_____

_____

_____

_____

_____

My Exercise Log

You can print this page out and use it daily or weekly to track your exercise progress.

Exercise: _____

Time Spent: _____

Miles (if applicable): _____

How did you feel before exercising?

_____

_____

_____

How do you feel afterwards?

_____

_____

_____

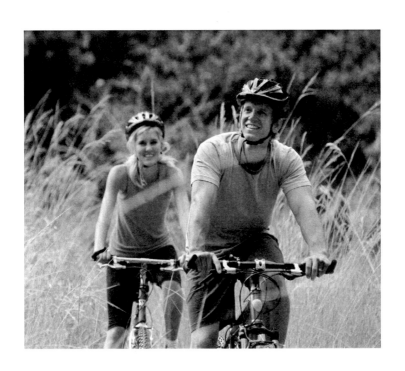

Reflections

What did you learn this week on the Alkaline Lifestyle?

_____

_____

_____

_____

How are you feeling about your healthy transformation?

_____

_____

_____

_____

What changes are you making this week?

_____

_____

_____

Do you have any questions? Write them below, then go to **www.alkalinelifestyle.com** and ask the experts.

_____

_____

_____

Action Steps

This week, I will take the following action steps to incorporate the Alkaline Lifestyle information into my daily routine:

1._____

2._____

3._____

4._____

5._____

6._____

7._____

8._____

Weekly Check In

Today's date:_____

My height:_____

My current weight:_____

My BMI:_____

My pH today:_____

The optimal range is 6.8 to 7.2._____

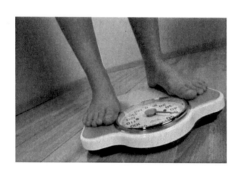

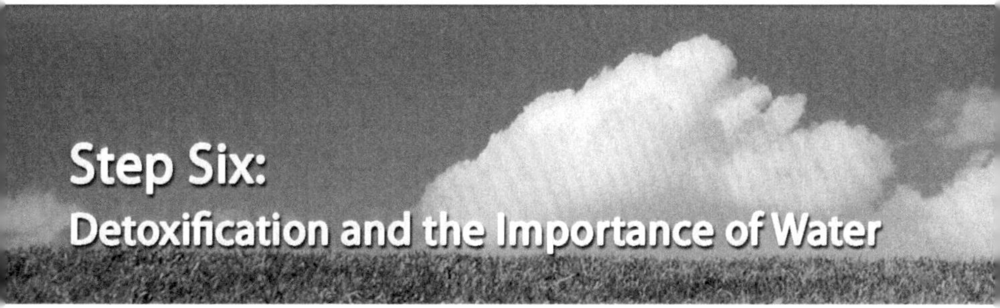

Step Six:
Detoxification and the Importance of Water

Detoxification helps your body shed the accumulated toxins that an acidic condition encourages the body to store. Simple detoxification methods can be used at home. Ionized alkaline mineral water aids detoxification, overall alkalinity, and health.

Are you overweight? If so, your body may have stored toxins in the fat tissues. How do you feel about this?

_____

_____

_____

Can you participate in a juice fast?

_____

_____

What steps can you take for detoxification?

_____

_____

_____

_____

How much water do you drink each day?

_____

How can you increase your water intake if you need to?

_____

_____

_____

Have you had your water tested? If so – what were the results?

_____

_____

_____

Can you invest in either a water filtration system or an ionized alkaline water machine?

_____

_____

_____

_____

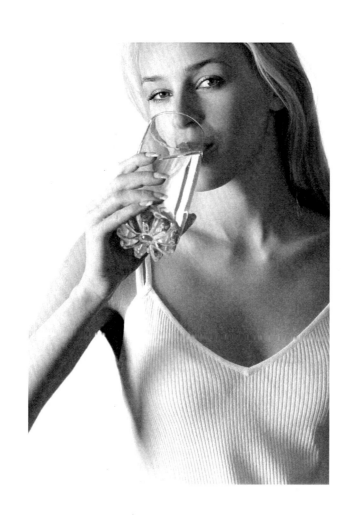

Reflections

What did you learn this week on the Alkaline Lifestyle?

_____

_____

_____

_____

How are you feeling about your healthy transformation?

_____

_____

_____

_____

What changes are you making this week?

_____

_____

_____

Do you have any questions? Write them below, then go to **www.alkalinelifestyle.com** and ask the experts.

_____

_____

_____

Action Steps

This week, I will take the following action steps to incorporate the Alkaline Lifestyle information into my daily routine:

1._____

2._____

3._____

4._____

5._____

6._____

7._____

8._____

Weekly Check In

Today's date:_____

My height:_____

My current weight:_____

My BMI:_____

My pH today:_____

The optimal range is 6.8 to 7.2._____

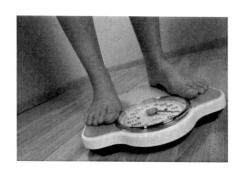

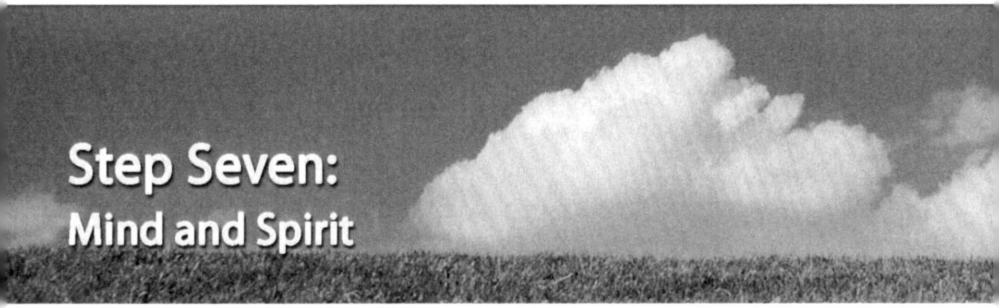

Step Seven:
Mind and Spirit

The Alkaline Lifestyle includes methods of creating a positive, peaceful mindset. This includes positive thinking and methods to connect with creativity. The Mind and Spirit book will include more exercises and ideas on this topic, but this section of the Journal and Workbook will get you started.

Do you consider yourself an optimist or a pessimist?

_____

_____

_____

Do you recognize your internal chatter, the monologue that runs through your head? Sometimes it goes by so quickly that it's tough to identify. If you can hear it, what's the general tone – negative, critical, positive?

_____

_____

_____

Everyone has negative, critical and judgmental thoughts from time to time. How can you transform them?

_____

_____

_____

_____

_____

Affirmations are positive statements you repeat to yourself to reprogram your internal 'tape' so that it 'plays' positive messages. Louise Hay, one of the foremost thinkers in positive affirmations, says that the two most important ones are –

I love myself.

I approve of myself.

Can you imagine yourself saying those statements? Try repeating them silently to yourself.

Affirmations are positive statements written in the present tense. You can create your own affirmations based on the goals that you set for yourself at the start of this Journal and Workbook.

Write several affirmation statements here:

_____

_____

_____

_____

An example:

I now weight 150 pounds.

I can run a mile without stopping.

I love my body

I love eating healthy, alkaline foods.

I am healthy.

I will only think positive thoughts.

Another important aspect of the Alkaline Lifestyle is connecting to your spiritual side. Many people find that nature helps them do this.

Do you enjoy time in nature?

_____

_____

_____

List your favorite places in nature to visit, such as the beach, the mountains, etc:

_____

_____

_____

_____

_____

_____

_____

Can you include more time in these places in your life?

_____

_____

_____

Search for 3 pictures of natural places that appeal to you. Print them and keep them at your desk or work space.

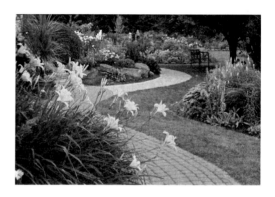

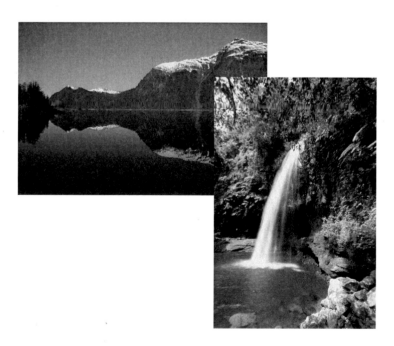

Another important aspect of the Alkaline Lifestyle is embracing your spiritual side through creativity. Creativity is not limited to the typical arts we think of such as drawing or painting. It may include....

Cooking
Fashion
Painting
Drawing
Sculpting
Knitting and needlecrafts
Miniatures
Dance
Listening to music
Playing a musical instrument
Creative writing
Crafts of all kinds
Creating Balloon characters for children
Model building
Games
Gardening
Fish keeping
Singing
Collecting
Playing with pets

Do you enjoy anything on the list on the previous page?

_____

_____

_____

_____

Do any of these ideas appeal to you?

_____

_____

_____

_____

_____

How can you include more creative play in your life?

_____

_____

_____

_____

_____

_____

Reflections

What did you learn this week on the Alkaline Lifestyle?

_____

_____

_____

_____

How are you feeling about your healthy transformation?

_____

_____

_____

_____

What changes are you making this week?

_____

_____

_____

Do you have any questions? Write them below, then go to **www.alkalinelifestyle.com** and ask the experts.

_____

_____

_____

Action Steps

This week, I will take the following action steps to incorporate the Alkaline Lifestyle information into my daily routine:

1._____

2._____

3._____

4._____

5._____

6._____

7._____

8._____

Weekly Check In

Today's date:_____

My height:_____

My current weight:_____

My BMI:_____

My pH today:_____

The optimal range is 6.8 to 7.2._____

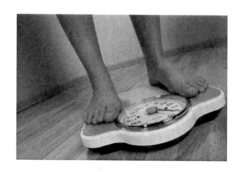

Step Eight:
Making Positive Changes Lasting Changes

You now have the basics of the Alkaline Lifestyle, presented Step by Step.

You know the foods to eat, the water to drink, the importance of exercise and detoxification. You understand the mind-spirit connection to the Alkaline Lifestyle.

How will you put it all together? Let's make a weekly Action Plan.

1. Pick one day of the week where you can spend a little bit of time planning and thinking. You don't need a lot of time. A few minutes will do.
2. Choose a small, simple goal for the week, such as increasing your intake of alkaline foods, remembering to take your supplements, increasing your exercise time or making room for creative play and meditation.
3. What steps do you need to take to achieve your goal? List them.
4. Look at your schedule for the week's activities. Are there any days when you will be eating out? Plan now for alkalizing on the go.
5. Write down your meal plan for the week – at least dinners. Make your shopping list now.
6. Write your exercise schedule down. If you place it on your calendar, you are more likely to stick with it.

Weekly Action Plan Template

Print as many of these pages off as you like for your personal use.

Week: (dates) _____

Special Events – Activities This Week:

_____

_____

_____

_____

_____

_____

Exercise Days and Activities:

_____

_____

_____

_____

_____

_____

My Weekly Goal is to:

_____

_____

_____

_____

I will take the following steps to achieve this goal:

_____

_____

_____

_____

_____

Here are the alkaline meals I've chosen for this week:

_____

_____

_____

_____

_____

_____

My shopping list – make sure I have on hand the following:

_____
_____
_____
_____
_____
_____
_____
_____
_____
_____
_____
_____
_____
_____
_____
_____

_____

CHECK IN – CELEBRATE SUCCESS

Look back at the very first list of goals you created at the start of this workbook.

How did you do?

_____

_____

_____

_____

How are you feeling about your progress?

_____

_____

_____

_____

_____

What else would you like to achieve?

_____

_____

_____

_____

_____

What questions do you have that we can answer for you?

_____

_____

_____

_____

_____

_____

What can you do to celebrate your success?

_____

_____

_____

_____

_____

_____

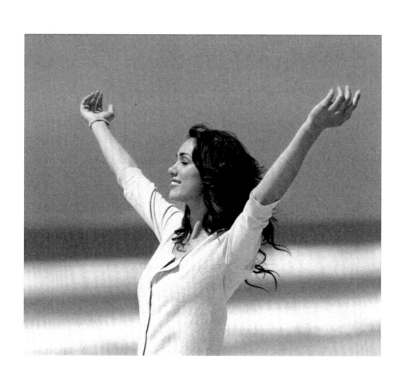

Journal and Workbook: Step by Step Transition Guide to the Alkaline Lifestyle
By the Editors, Staff, and Experts at AlkalineLifestyle.com

Published by Alkaline People Publishing
6352 Corte Del Abeto, Suite H
Carlsbad, CA 92011
888.800.0459
www.AlkalinePeoplePublishing.com

Printed in the United States
1st Printing January 2011

THE AMERICAN INDIAN IN AMERICA

Volume I

This Book Belongs To:

Thomas Monet Richardson

The American Indian in America is a two-volume survey of the history of the American Indian. Volume II traces Indian history from the early 19th century to the present.

The IN AMERICA *Series*

THE **AMERICAN INDIAN** IN AMERICA

Volume I

JAYNE CLARK JONES

Published by
Lerner Publications Company
Minneapolis, Minnesota

ACKNOWLEDGMENTS

The illustrations are reproduced through the courtesy of: pp. 6, 16 (bottom), 27, 48, 67, 75, Museum of the American Indian, Heye Foundation; pp. 8, 23, 78, 80, 85, 94, Independent Picture Service; pp. 11, 81, United States Department of the Interior; p. 13, Field Museum of Natural History, by Charles R. Knight; p. 14, Denver Museum of Natural History; p. 16 (top), Southwest Museum; p. 18, Robert S. Peabody Foundation for Archaeology; p. 19, Mexican Government Tourism Department; pp. 21 (left), 31, 54, 55, 71, 74, Smithsonian Institution; pp. 21 (right), 44, National Museums of Canada; p. 25, Thomas Gilcrease Institute of American History and Art; pp. 28, 59, Peabody Museum, Harvard University; p. 29, Brooklyn Museum; pp. 33, 40, 47, 51, 62, 63 (left), 72, American Museum of Natural History; p. 35 (left), Historical Society of Pennsylvania; p. 35 (right), J.J. Hill Library, Saint Paul; p. 37, The Corcoran Gallery of Art; pp. 22, 39, 52, 60, 63 (right), Royal Ontario Museum, Canada; p. 43, National Museum, Copenhagen; p. 57, The Museum of Fine Arts, Houston; p. 64, New York State Museum and Science Service; p. 65, New York Public Library, Rare Book Division, Astor, Lenox and Tilden Foundations; p. 69, Travel Division, South Dakota Department of Highways; p. 77, The Albertina, Vienna; p. 83, The Mansell Collection; p. 84, Virginia State Library; pp. 88, 91, 97, Library of Congress; p. 95, Religious News Service; p. 98, Detroit Historical Museum.

Front cover illustrations: "The Last of the Buffalo" by Albert Bierstadt, The Corcoran Gallery of Art (top); "Indian Encampment on Lake Huron" by Paul Kane, The Art Gallery of Toronto (bottom); "Chief Iron Shirt" by Karl Bodmer (insert). Back cover illustration: "In Front of the Chief's Tent" by Karl Bodmer. Library Edition

LIBRARY OF CONGRESS CATALOGING IN PUBLICATION DATA

Jones, Jayne Clark.
The American Indian in America.

(The In America Series)
SUMMARY: Two volumes survey the American Indian from prehistory through the twentieth century, including discussions of his origin, culture, the impact of white civilization on his society, and Amerindian contributions to United States history and culture.

1. Indians of North America—Juvenile literature. [1. Indians of North America] I. Title.

E77.4.J66   970.1   73-3378
ISBN 0-8225-0224-0 [Library] v. 1
ISBN 0-8225-1001-4 [Paper] v. 1

International Standard Book Number: 0-8225-0224-0 Library Edition
International Standard Book Number: 0-8225-1001-4 Paper Edition

Library of Congress Catalog Card Number: 73-3378

8 9 10 90 89 88 87 86 85

. . . CONTENTS . . .

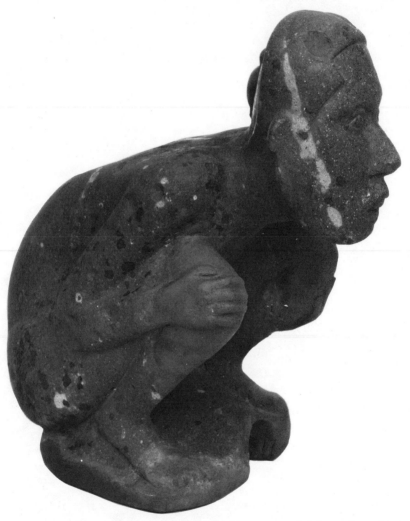

Ancient art objects often serve as a valuable source of information about Indian prehistory. This "squatting man" pipe, made by Indians of the prehistoric mound-building culture, was probably used for ceremonial purposes.

PART I

Prehistory
and Amerindian Culture

1. *What Is Prehistory?*

There are no other stories like this one "in America." The American Indians are not one but many peoples with many cultures. In this they are not unlike the white men of Europe, who are divided into nations, each with an ancestral homeland, history, and tradition that live on in new times and new homes. There has been hate, mistrust, and war among the American Indians, but there is also much that they have in common, many similarities among them, and much that they share. Perhaps the brief outline in these small books will induce the reader to look further into the vast and complicated subject of America's Indian heritage.

Generations of red men have occupied this land, time out of mind. They are the native Americans. Yet, like everyone else in this nation of immigrants, they are the descendants of people who came here from somewhere else, and their history, like that of white Americans, begins in 1492.

A *history* of any group of people is an account of past events based on written records. If the records are too few or of the wrong kind, the account may be pieced out with other kinds of information based on material things that may have survived from the time in question—buildings, coins, pottery, paintings. If there are no written records at all and only material remains can be studied, we enter the realm of *prehistory*.

Most Americans of Pre-Columbian times had no written records. Though hundreds of native languages were spoken in the North American continent when Europeans arrived, only a few groups in Mexico and Guatemala had devised systems of writing. In tribes without systems of writing, a man could record his war deeds in a picture story painted on a hide. A totem pole could be carved to suggest a brief family history. However, most tribal history was preserved in songs, stories, and recollections that were passed orally from one generation to another. An historian must treat such material as folklore unless he can verify it in some way.

Little of the history of any American society before the arrival of Columbus is known to us. Therefore, because we cannot

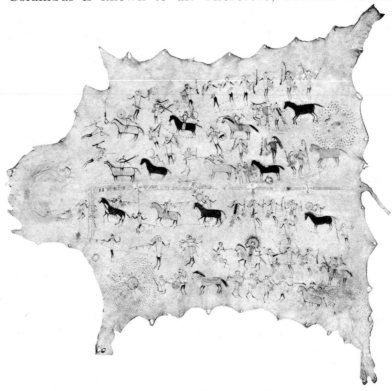

Indians who had no system of writing often painted picture stories on animal hides as a means of keeping records.

speak of dates, personalities, or events, we must content ourselves with describing cultures, societies, and their development. A *society* is a group of people living together and sharing a common *culture*, or way of life. Anything that a person makes or uses to maintain or enhance his life is part of his culture and is called a *culture trait*. A culture with many traits is said to be more "complex" than one with a few.

There is one problem that men of all societies and cultures share—what they are to eat, and how they are to get it. The way a man gets his living is called his *mode of subsistence*, and the rest of his culture is organized around it. A man who gets all he needs with a stick and a knife has a less complex material culture than a man who uses a bow and arrows, spear, nets, traps, hooks, and harpoons in his food quest.

A very complex culture implies a large society. When a culture becomes so complex and a society so large that it must organize itself in order to continue, it may reach a cultural stage called *civilization*. A civilization will usually have several, but not necessarily all, of the following characteristics: city life, a high degree of social and economic organization, bureaucratic government, monumental art and architecture, and a system of writing. In the Western Hemisphere the Olmecs, Zapotecs, Mayas, and Aztecs of Mexico, and the Incas of Peru attained civilization in Pre-Columbian times.

Cultures change because the needs, habits, or ideas of people change. Some changes come rather easily and quickly, but language, family relationships, burial customs, and diet are so fixed by habit, custom, and prejudice that only some great disturbance will cause a sudden change. Otherwise, people do things each day pretty much as they did them the day before.

Because the lives of people do not change much from day to day, scientists can learn a great deal by studying the material objects used in everyday life. Hidden in the soil near places where people have lived or camped are things they have thrown away, buried, or left behind. Beginning with those things nearest the surface, archaeologists carefully uncover the objects where they are found. The items are mapped, picked up, labeled, and identified, if possible. Layer after layer of soil is removed, sometimes with a shovel, sometimes with a teaspoon, until a point is reached where there is no further sign of human life. Finally, in what looks like a collection of old trash, anthropologists and other specialists look for the answers to their questions. These are the clues from which we must try to reconstruct the cultures of Pre-Columbian America.

Many scientists play a role in the study of American prehistory. Geologists can tell if the land has changed since people lived there. Paleontologists can study human bones and describe the way the people looked. Bones and shells from rubbish heaps reveal what animals they hunted and ate. From samples of the soil, paleobotanists sort out pollen and seeds which show not only what plants were eaten but whether they were wild or domestic, and exactly what the varieties were. Laboratory tests can tell roughly how old the organic materials are. In this way, the skills of many experts are used to build a picture of the people who lived in one locality and the way their life changed over the centuries.

Most of those who have studied Indian prehistory (and history as well) have been white men. The information in most books about Indians answers questions that white men think are important enough to ask. It is white men who arrange cultures from simple to complex, with civilization at the top. People are apt to assume that a culture which uses guns and snowmobiles is not only more complex but "more advanced" than one that uses harpoons and sleds. In other words, the values of white civilization are written into its descriptions and accounts of nonwhite people.

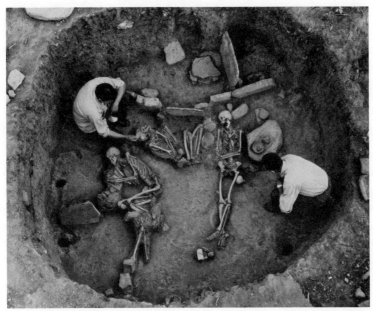

Archaeologists carefully uncover human bones and artifacts at Mesa Verde, Colorado, a site inhabited by Indians in prehistoric times.

It is important to be aware that there is much in both Indian prehistory and history that we do not know, much we know that we do not understand, much that we misunderstand. And, equally important, we should realize that it is possible to make use of the information that has been assembled without accepting the assumptions and conclusions that go with it. Everyone must decide for himself whether or not "more complex" means "higher," or "more advanced" means "better."

2. *The Paleo-Indians*

For 70,000 or 80,000 years the last great glacier of the Ice Age, the Wisconsin, covered most of North America, advancing as far south as Iowa and Missouri. The Wisconsin Glacier advanced and retreated several times before the Ice Age finally came to an end about 9000 B.C. At its maximum, about one-third of the world's surface water was collected in this sheet of ice, which reached a depth of two miles in places. With so much water held in the form of ice and snow, the sea level was 150 to 300 feet lower than it is today. A number of places on earth now separated by narrow, shallow strips of sea were joined by dry land. It would have been possible at that time for men and animals to walk from Malaya to Java and Sumatra, or from France to England, or from Siberia to Alaska—and that is most certainly what they did do.

Bones turned to stone (fossils) help us follow the migrations of the Ice Age, or Pleistocene, mammals from the Old World to the New. These mammals, the great, grass-eating ancestors of so

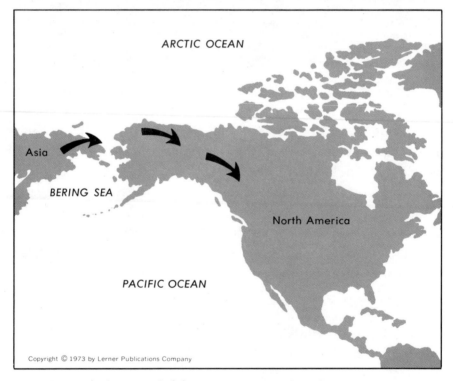

During the last period of the Ice Age, Asia and North America were joined by a narrow strip of dry land. Across this land bridge, the ancestors of the American Indians migrated to the New World.

many modern species, included the woolly rhinoceros, the mammoth, the mastodon, the giant sloth, the Ice Age camel, and the ancestors of modern horses. When these great grazing and browsing animals moved, following the rich grassy plains east of the Rocky Mountains down from the north into the United States, the meat eaters followed—hyena-like dogs, saber-toothed cats, and man.

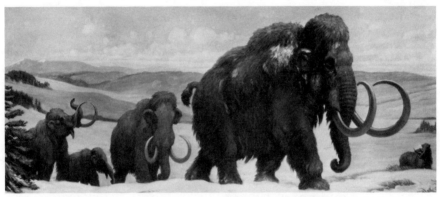

The mastodon was one of the large grass-eating mammals that migrated from the Old World to the New World during the Ice Age.

When the glacier receded, as it did several times, the climate moderated, and the run-off from the melting glacier collected in great lakes and marshes. The southwestern plains and the Great Basin, which are hot and arid now, were cool, moist grasslands then, a perfect environment for big game animals. These animals were what the first immigrants to America were looking for.

By 10,000 B.C., men had established themselves throughout the rich and diverse North American continent. They had brought with them fire, language, the ability to make tools and weapons of stone, and a culture based on hunting. There is some evidence that others may have come even earlier—men who had not yet learned to make stone dart points. Certainly others came later— the Eskimos, for instance—until finally the sea rose and blocked the way. These earliest Americans are sometimes called *Paleo-Indians*. They are the ancestors of the American Indians of historic times.

The oldest known culture in North America is called the *Big-Game Hunting Tradition*. The hunters of big game were necessarily nomads. They hunted the giant Ice Age animals with large projectile points well designed for their supersized prey. At many camp and kill sites across the United States, expertly made stone lance or dart points have been found in place among the bones of animals that are now extinct. These early men had other good stone tools as well—thin, sharp knives, scrapers for preparing animal hides and carcasses, drills and sandstone "smoothers" for smoothing stone, bone, and wood objects. A few bone tools have also been found—scrapers, awls, and needles with eyes. These are evidence that the Big-Game Hunters depended on game for hides and other animal products as well as for food. Except for the caves where many of these things have been found, no trace of any kind of shelter survives. But living in the cool, wet glacial climate, the Big-Game Hunters doubtless did have both shelter and warm clothing.

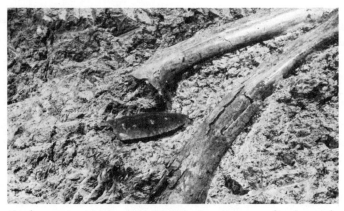

Man's presence in America 10,000 years ago was firmly established in 1927, when this spear point was discovered among the bones of an Ice Age bison at Folsom, New Mexico.

About 8000 B.C. a warmer period began. In the Southwest the glacial waters slowly dried up, leaving behind salty ponds and swamps or alkaline flatlands. The lush grasses faded. Those plants that survived adapted to an ever decreasing water supply. Since about 2500 B.C. the climate of the United States has been as it is now. Except for the coastal regions and the higher elevations in the mountains, the western half of the country became a desert. The giant Pleistocene grazing animals either perished or followed the retreating grasslands. The Big-Game Hunters followed them into river valleys, onto the high plains where grass remained, and into the well-watered woodlands east of the Mississippi.

Plants, animals, and people who stayed in desert regions changed over the generations as the climate changed. People had to depend more on gathering wild plant foods and less on hunting. By 8000 or 7000 B.C. a second ancient American culture had developed in response to the problems of desert life. It is known as the *Desert Tradition.*

Dry caves in Utah, Nevada, Arizona, and southern Oregon are the sites of many finds from the Desert Tradition. Because of the extreme dryness of the desert climate, even perishable plant and animal materials are preserved so that we have a much fuller picture of desert life than we do that of the Big-Game Hunters. By studying these desert finds, scientists are able to describe the projectiles used before bows and arrows. The smaller game of the desert required smaller stone points than the big game. Darts, made by attaching the stone point to a wooden shaft, were propelled toward the target with the help of a wooden throwing stick (atlatl).

Also essential to the desert way of life were stone grinding tools. The *mano*, a handstone for grinding plant foods, and the *metate*, a stone slab that provides the surface against which the food is ground, are characteristic finds at desert sites. From plant

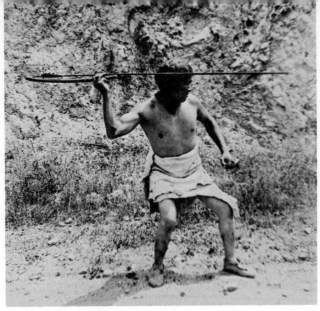

A modern Indian demonstrates the use of the ancient atlatl, a wooden spear-thrower used before the development of the bow and arrow.

fibers of many kinds the desert dwellers made baskets for gathering and storage, sandals, mats, cordage, and nets for catching small animals. It is miraculous that so many fragments of these things are still intact 10,000 years after they were made.

In contrast to the immense tracts of desert is the narrow strip along the northern Pacific coast of North America. The wooded mountains, the rivers, and the sea make this an area of amazing riches. Perhaps as long ago as 9000 B.C. a third Paleo-Indian culture known as the *Old Cordilleran Tradition* had developed in this environment. There are sites of Old Cordilleran habitation near rapids on the Columbia and Fraser rivers of the Northwest. These locations are great fishing spots even today. The ancient settlements were probably permanent fishing camps. Bones of

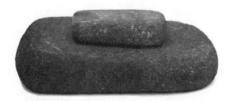

Indians of the prehistoric Desert Tradition used the mano (top) and metate (bottom) to grind plant foods.

sea mammals, fish, and game are all found on these spots, along with some implements unknown to the Big-Game and Desert people. Old Cordilleran dart points have a characteristic willow-leaf shape and are smaller than Big-Game points. Other implements found at Old Cordilleran sites include harpoons made of bone and antler for the hunting of sea mammals, hooks for fishing, knives of slate, and other stone woodworking tools. These people were clearly less specialized than the Big-Game Hunters. They went hunting along the coast for sea mammals and in the mountains for game but seem to have returned with the kill to the riverside settlements. Fish, particularly salmon, was an important element in their subsistence.

To explain the cultures of many of the American Indian tribes as they were when the white men came, one more mode of subsistence must be added to those of the Paleo-Indians. In the arid highlands of central Mexico, people who were following a desert way of life about 10,000 B.C. began to gather the seeds of certain native grasses. These grasses were the earliest ancestors of maize, or corn, the staple grain of the New World. Once again the evidence of centuries of change has been found in dry caves that were used as shelter by countless generations.

The tiny ears of wild corn, about half an inch in length, bore a tassel, relatively few kernels, and a husk of only two leaves, which did not interfere with the release of mature seeds. Ears of domestic corn are completely covered by a tough husk that makes it impossible for the seeds to scatter without the help of man. Between the two types are centuries of cultivation and cross-breeding; the process began between 7000 and 5000 B.C.

The idea of protecting and then actually planting and cultivating desirable food plants must have developed in more than one place during this period. Some of the people who were gathering wild corn, wild beans, and chili peppers were cultivating and eating domestic squash and avocados at the same

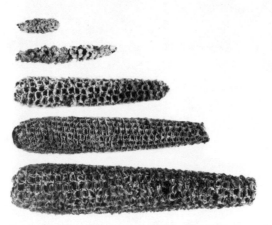

This collection of corncobs shows the evolution of corn from its earliest stage to its modern form. Wild corn (top) was domesticated in Mexico sometime before 5000 B.C. Modern corn (bottom) did not appear until 5,000 years later.

time. Of the wide variety of native plants that the people of Mexico brought under cultivation, three—corn, beans, and squash—became the basic crops of North America.

Agriculture makes it necessary for people to stay put somewhere near their crops, at least during the growing season. In this way, village life begins. Villages existed in Mexico by 3000 B.C. By 2300 B.C. pottery, another culture trait associated with agriculture and sedentary life, had appeared. Earlier, between 5200 and 3400 B.C., many plants were domesticated—corn, gourds, chili peppers, squashes, and several kinds of beans. At first, domestic plants accounted for only 10 percent of the food supply. During the period when people began to live in settlements of permanent houses and make pottery, 30 percent of their food supply came from domestic plants. The ears of corn became much larger, and cotton was added to the list of domestic plants.

The civilizations of Mexico developed on the foundation of the agricultural village economy. After 850 B.C. people were irrigating their crops, and the population had increased. Temples were built on the tops of huge mounds, and religious centers grew up around them. By the time of Christ, the temple complexes had become true cities. The ears of corn had become fully modern, and the people derived 85 percent of their food from agriculture. The reliable food supply provided by agriculture allowed part of the population to pursue other activities. The magnificent cities with their carefully arranged pyramids, streets, plazas, and ball courts could not have come into being without planning and organized labor on a gigantic scale. Beautiful textiles, pottery, ornaments, and decorations of precious metals, stone, plaster, and mural art were the result of skills developed and refined over long periods of time. The influence of these achievements spread like waves from Mexico and helped shape the cultures of many of the native people of the United States.

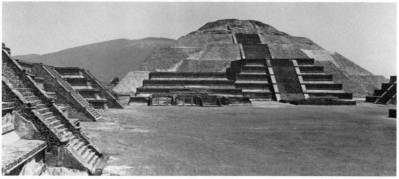

The Pyramid of the Moon at the city of Teotihuacán in central Mexico. In the period between 300 and 700 A.D., Teotihuacán covered an area of nearly seven square miles and was inhabited by 50,000 people.

3. *Amerindian Culture*

At the time when the Paleo-Indians broke away from their Asian relatives, the races of man were not yet as distinctly different as they are today. Each group of immigrants developed separately and differently. There are still physical resemblances between Indians and Asians, but the natives of the Western Hemisphere belong to a separate race. Migrants whose ancestors

came at a later time—the Athabaskans and the Eskimos—
resemble the Mongolian peoples more closely than do other
American Indians. But all American Indians have developed
their racial identity in the New World.

The Paleo-Indian cultures and later ones that developed from
them are the results of adaptations to different environments.
Environmental differences made certain cultural changes possible, others necessary. The climate and resources of the land
set the limits of what any man can do. No one will be a farmer
in the Arctic or hunt whales in North Dakota. Woodworking will
not be a highly developed art in Arizona, nor will houses be made
of adobe on Puget Sound. But contact with new people will
suggest new ideas, new objects, and new ways to use them.
Moreover, of the choices of methods, ideas, and resources available in every region, many different combinations are possible.
American Indian cultures demonstrate the fascinating variety of
these combinations.

A good many culture traits, both material and nonmaterial,
are common to so many Indian groups that they can be regarded
as *Amerindian*. Many of these traits are shared by cultures that
are very different in other ways. No two groups make or use these
things in exactly the same way. Nevertheless, these shared
culture traits can be regarded as the common store of Indian
culture.

Material Culture

All Indians hunted whatever animals their surroundings
offered. The universal weapons were the lance, and the bow and
arrow. Bows and arrows began to replace the dart and atlatl
about 500 A.D. By the time of contact with the white man, they
were used throughout the continent.

Nearly all tribes gathered a variety of wild plant foods. All
those Indians who practiced agriculture raised corn. Others were

familiar with it through trade even though they did not grow it themselves. The use of tobacco, a native American plant, probably began in Mexico and spread throughout most of the United States. Tobacco was raised by some people who did no other gardening at all. Where it was not grown it was sometimes obtained by trade. It was used in several ways but was most commonly smoked for ceremonial purposes.

All Indians preserved some of their food by drying it. Stone-boiling, a very ancient method of cooking food by dropping hot stones into water until it boiled, seems to have been widely known. Some Indians, however, used it only on trips or in emergencies. Basketry of some kind and pottery was made by most Indians. All made at least some items of clothing from animal hides. The breechclout was the standard garment for men almost everywhere. (The breechclout was a strip of cloth or hide passed between the legs and held in place by a rope or thong tied at the waist.) From the earliest times Indians kindled their fires with a fire drill. A bow was used to spin a hardwood drill into a soft wooden block until the friction produced a flame.

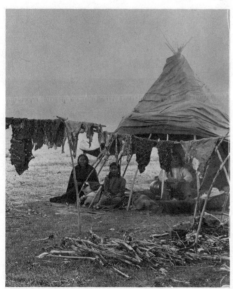 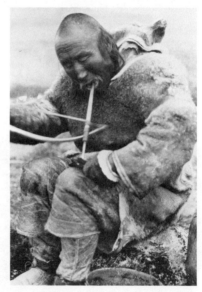

The customs of preserving food by drying (left) and of kindling fires with a fire drill (right) are two culture traits common to many groups of American Indians.

Round shelters made of several poles joined at the top to form a cone or bent over to form a dome shape were familiar to most Indians. Even where permanent housing was of some other kind, temporary or portable housing for hunting or gathering trips was often such a pole structure covered with bark, hides, mats, or brush.

Most goods were transported on the backs of men. In America a strap called a *tumpline* was attached to the load and worn across the forehead. Dogs, everywhere the ancient companions of man, were one of the few domestic animals in North America. They pulled loads, carried things, and hunted for their masters. They were also eaten, sheared for their wool, sacrificed, and loved as pets.

Most Indian babies were tied to cradleboards of some kind until they were old enough to walk. In this device a child could be conveniently transported and "parked" near his mother at all times. Mothers often carried these cradleboards by means of a tumpline.

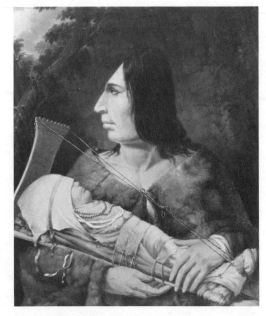

A woman of the Flathead tribe uses a cradleboard to carry her child.

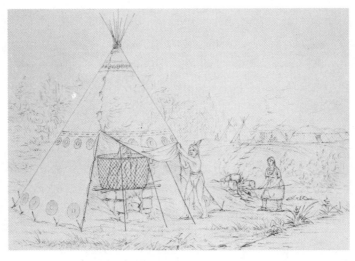

This sketch by George Catlin pictures the custom of sweating as it was practiced among the Mandan Indians of the Missouri Valley.

Sweating was practiced by American Indians from the Arctic to the Rio Grande. Special sweathouses were superheated with either dry heat or steam. The people inside stood it as long as possible and then took a sudden dip in the nearest stream or lake. Sweating was practiced as a means of producing a feeling of well-being, as a treatment for disease, and as a religious purification.

Nonmaterial Culture

Most readers will be familiar with the brief list of the material culture traits shared by native Americans. However, the nonmaterial life of the people who used these objects is far harder to describe. What did the Indian societies value? What did they regard as good and just? How did they organize and govern themselves? What did they fear? What did they do for fun? Each Indian culture today can find Indian identity in these nonmaterial things even though the bows and arrows, tipis, and cradleboards are gone. Amerindian values and traditions are of lasting importance to both native and white Americans.

Language

In the center of any culture is its language, and Indian languages show as much variety as any other aspect of Indian life. At least 200 separate languages were spoken in Pre-Columbian America north of Mexico. Many of these languages have disappeared, but over 50 are still spoken as the mother tongues of Indians living today.

Linguists believe that families of related Indian languages developed from the languages spoken by each ancient group of immigrants. When one of the original bands divided, the language of each new group began to develop differently. All languages change as time passes. New objects and ideas call for new words and expressions. New words can be made up out of two or more old words, or they can be borrowed, along with the things they name, from other people. Pronunciations also change, but they change very slowly and by degrees. At some time before two groups originally speaking the same language have been separated by too much time and distance, their speech will have become different, but they will still be able to understand each other. At this point we say that each group speaks a different *dialect* of the same language. Eventually they will no longer be able to understand each other at all, even though they began with the same language. Whenever either group divides again, the process is repeated. It is this process of division and change over thousands of years that has produced the amazing number of mutually unintelligible American Indian languages. Languages being spoken today can still be sorted into families by language experts who can detect traces of their original relationships.

For American Indians, language has a unique function and importance. Although Indian languages differed greatly, most Indians shared a special attitude toward language and its use. Without writing, tribal traditions of law, religion, history, and poetry had to be passed orally from one generation to the next.

Government was carried on in public meetings. Chiefs kept their power, in many cases, only as long as they could persuade others to support them. In council meetings every member could express his point of view before a decision was made. Chiefs often had speakers who could put their ideas into correct and fine-sounding language. Warriors told about their exploits at public meetings. Storytellers were revered members of the community, and a favorite Indian pastime was listening to stories. In all of these activities, skill in oratory—elegant, correct, and moving expression—was highly prized and admired.

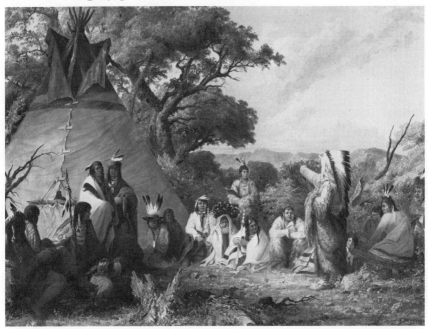

Indian skill in oratory was often put to good use in council meetings such as the one shown in this painting by Seth Eastman.

Social Organization and Kinship

A most important and persistent nonmaterial trait of any society is its system of social organization and the relationships it recognizes. Both Indian and white society use the family as the basic social unit. Parents living with their unmarried children, a *nuclear family*, is the most familiar form of family in white society. When parents, unmarried and married children, grandchildren, and an occasional single or aged aunt or uncle live together and share their economic life, the unit is called an *extended family*. An extended family may live in one large house, or related nuclear families may live close to their relatives and share the work and income of the larger unit. The extended family was the most common kind of family unit throughout North America.

A family may pass its identity (its name, property, social status) through either the male or the female side of the family, or through both. When the inheritance is passed through one side, all the members of the family who receive the inheritance are part of a *lineage*. If the maternal side carries the family name, the mother, her children, her daughter's children, and her granddaughter's children are all members of her lineage. If the lineage is the basis for an extended family, then a woman's daughters bring their husbands to the maternal home when they marry, and their children become part of the *matrilineage*. A son, on the other hand, leaves his mother's home when he marries. He lives with his wife's people, and his children belong to her lineage, not to his. The reverse is true in a *patrilineage*, which is based on a system of paternal descent. Some tribes traced descent from both parents. When they married they might join either side of the family, or neither, if they preferred.

Two other larger social groups widely found among Indian societies are the clan and the moiety. The *clan* is a kind of artificial family made up of two or more lineages who believe that they are related through some mythical ancestor. The ancestor is often some superanimal such as the raven, wolf, bear, or buffalo. That animal has special importance for the clan and is called its *totem*. Members of the Wolf clan might feel that they share some of the qualities of the wolf, that wolves are their particular protectors, that some part of a wolf—say, its teeth or tail—is especially lucky as a charm. Clans also have names of other kinds —Wind, Thunder, Sore-lip, Gray-eye—but these clans also usually have a totem. Every clan bestows certain privileges and imposes responsibilities on its members.

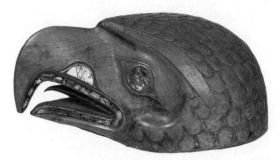

An eagle headdress worn by the chief of the Eagle Clan in the Niska tribe of the Northwest Coast

In American Indian societies, clan membership was inherited and could not be changed. Personal names usually carried clan identification. Since clan members believed themselves to be related, they were usually required to marry outside their own clan. Everyone had the duty of kinship toward his fellow clan members, and each clan had both social responsibilities and social privileges. A clansman could expect help and hospitality from fellow members and, in time of trouble, he could call on them for assistance. It was the duty of the clan, for instance, to seek revenge if one of its members was murdered. Two clans might assist at childbirths, arrange funerals, or help build houses for each other. A clan might also be required to perform some service for the whole tribe, such as sponsoring a particular religious celebration or caring for a sacred object. A clan's special privilege might be the exclusive right to use a certain hunting or fishing spot, or to provide a particular tribal officer.

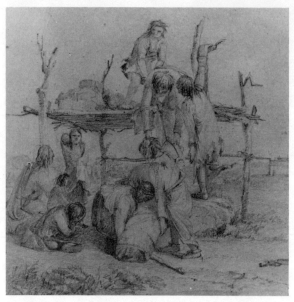

Clans often had the responsibility of assisting at the burials of members of other clans.

The *moiety*, another social grouping found all over North America, is a division of the tribe or band into two halves (*moieté* means half in French). Some tribes had both clans and moieties, some had only one of the two, a few had neither. Moiety membership might be determined by inheritance, by order of birth, or by season of birth. Moiety names sometimes emphasized the idea of opposites—Summer and Winter, or Peace and War. The Creek War Moiety always supported the war party in tribal councils, while the Peace Moiety argued for peace. The Pawnee Summer Moiety always camped and sat on the south side of any site where the people gathered, while the Winter people took places on the north. Eskimos of the Baffin Islands born in spring and summer belong to the Duck Moiety; those born in fall and winter, to the Ptarmigan Moiety. Moieties often have totems, as clans do. Where moieties were strong they functioned in the same way that clans did. Thus an individual usually married outside his own moiety. In other cases, as among the Eskimos, moieties simply offered a way of dividing the people into opposing sides for games or contests, or for a kind of good-natured, joking rivalry.

The term *tribe* usually refers to a group of people who share the same language and culture and identify with a particular territory or homeland. The American tribes had all kinds of political organization, ranging from very simple to very complex. A tribe may have been divided most of the time into bands or villages, without any tribal government. But most groups recognized their tribal affiliation at various times, for instance, when everyone gathered for a special hunt or ceremonial.

The tribes used the social institutions—lineage, clan, moiety (and some others)—in a variety of ways, but the principle of organization in Indian society was kinship rather than citizenship as it is in white society. The result was that, compared to most white Americans, Indians were members of larger family units and shared food, belongings, and social responsibility freely with a larger circle of relatives.

In spite of the difficulty and harshness of the life of many Indian societies, all Indians treated their young children with gentleness and affection. Even people who had very few material possessions themselves made toys for their children—dolls, tiny pots, miniature weapons, tools and canoes, balls, hoops and game

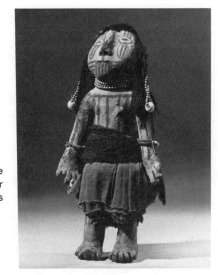

A pottery doll made by the Mojave Indians of Arizona. Dolls and other toys were given to Indian children as tokens of affection.

pieces, and little model animals. At least until the age of seven, children lived with a minimum of restrictions or discipline. They learned about their future as adults by watching and imitating their elders, and they were given very little formal instruction. The responsibilities of adulthood came eventually, however, and sometimes the passage into adult life was a difficult test, especially for boys. But during their early years, children were shielded and indulged as much as possible.

Indian attitudes toward ownership, which played such a crucial part in their dealings with white men, were closely related to their social system and to their world view. Indians saw the resources of life—land, air, and water—as unownable. Each tribe, however, occupied a territory as its own hunting ground and expected to keep it free from trespassers. The territory belonged to them in the same sense that the United States belongs to all Americans. However, strangers who were traveling or who were displaced from their own lands, as many were in later times, were often allowed to share it. Even tribes that wandered over vast areas regarded some spot as sacred because it was their place of origin, their tribal burial ground, or their ceremonial gathering place.

An Indian owned, that is, could do anything he liked with, his personal possessions—tools, weapons, clothing, and sometimes his individual dwelling. Often the game he killed and the crops he grew might have to be shared with others in the family or community. A family or clan might have the hereditary use of a particular field, fishing spot, or trapping place. An individual would inherit this right through his lineage, but he could not dispose of it in return for a payment of any kind because it belonged as much to his family and his descendants as it did to him. He *could* allow others to use his privilege or not as he pleased.

Indian society regulated itself without the use of prisons, written laws, or, for the most part, police, courts, or judges. When

Indians broke the rules of their society they were disciplined in a variety of ways. Misbehavior such as boasting or laziness was treated with public ridicule. Sometimes an offender was shamed into improvement by a public scolding from some older person. However, no one ever received public punishment from a member of his own family. Inappropriate behavior, especially in children, was treated with silence, a kind of rejection that was felt as punishment.

For crimes such as murder and adultery the relatives of the victim, members of either his family or clan, took punishment of the criminal into their own hands. An adulterer might be beaten or mutilated. A typical penalty for murder was to kill the murderer or some member of his family. In many tribes the injured family could be persuaded to accept payment instead of the execution. Usually a chief or some important elder would mediate between the two families.

The Plains tribes used a police force during their large annual hunts to prevent any individual from spoiling the hunt for the

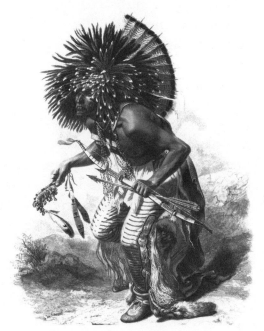

A member of the Hidatsa Dog Society, portrayed in an engraving by Karl Bodmer. The Dog Society served as a police force during the Hidatsa's annual hunts.

whole group. Anyone who frightened the game too early or who failed to follow hunt procedure could have his possessions destroyed or, in extreme cases, might even be killed.

In the Southeast and Southwest, town chiefs acted as judges. Certain other men were chosen to carry out the judgments. Most tribes regarded religious crimes, especially witchcraft, as the most serious of all crimes. Such offenses always received the severest penalties—physical punishment and death. On the whole, however, there was far less crime and far less punishment among Indians than among whites of the same period.

Religion and World View

The conditions of life were similar for all natives of Pre-Columbian America. Indians lived every day in a world that is hidden from people in modern urban societies—the real, whole, natural world. Their intimate knowledge of the life-giving forces of earth, sun, and rain, their daily dependence on other living things, and their own weakness in the face of natural forces gave them a realistic view of man's place in the universe. Ideas that white men try to express in scientific terms—biosphere, ecosystem, balance of nature, food chain—were expressed by Indians in poetic and religious images. Indians understood and acknowledged that man does not control the forces that govern his life but that he lives best when he is in harmony with them. Man has a place, but so do other things. Even the mosquito and the louse live in the world and have power because they exist. The earth is a good provider—a good mother. If no one is greedy or careless, there is enough for all. For white men, security lies in stockpiling against the future. For Indians, security lies in the shared strength of his kin and the new gifts of each season. Indian religious practices reflect this world view.

The land could be bountiful, but there was always the possibility of scarcity. Most Indians were acquainted with want as well as

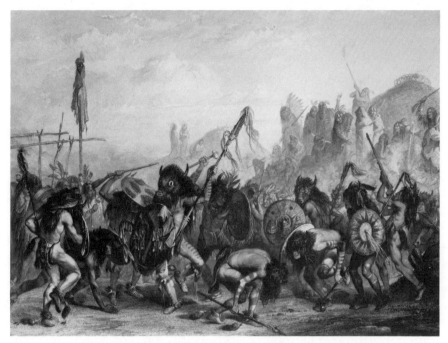

The Bison Dance of the Mandan Indians was a religious
ceremony that was performed to insure a successful hunt.

plenty. Every good thing in nature had an evil face as well. Rain
was needed for the corn to grow, but it might fall without stopping until the seed rotted in the ground or washed away in a
flood. The sun that brought the world to life in the spring could
also bring drought that withered everything green. The world
was not only wind, sun, hills, stones, plants, and animals but also
the force or spirit that made each thing behave in its own way.
Indian religion was based on the belief that this spirit world,
which exists alongside the visible world, made things happen for
either good or ill. But man could influence the behavior of the
spirits by not offending them, by being respectful, or by offering
suitable gifts.

Most tribes acknowledged one Great Spirit over all others.
They also believed in ghosts, which might be either good or harm-

ful. Most funeral rites were meant to keep the spirits of the dead from hurting the living or to speed those spirits on their way. To the extent that they believed in the spirits of the dead, all Indians believed in an afterlife. Most Indians had no systematic view of the spirit world or a belief in a hierarchy of spirits, but their world was full of unseen forces. People faced enemies, hunger, disease, and death at every hand. No man could expect to manage such superhuman problems without superhuman help.

Most Indians used a similar system for getting the spirit help they needed. A man or boy, often at puberty, would seek a spiritual meeting with some supernatural force. He would retire alone to a small hut in the woods or some other place apart. There he would fast and meditate until he saw or heard something, a dream or vision, that he could understand as a sign from a spirit. He might hear a wolf howling or dream of talking to a wolf, who taught him some magic. Whatever the experience, it was completely personal. The only proof that it happened at all lay in the benefits the individual received from the spirit. The benefits took many forms, but they were generally associated with the qualities of the animal spirit that bestowed them. The spirit helped in time of special need or gave some special knowledge or secret. The prayer, song, or ceremony taught by the spirit brought some spirit-power to the man who knew them. The deer spirit, for instance, could give a man the power to be a very successful deer hunter, to keep the deer out of the gardens, to run as swiftly as a deer, or to cure a particular disease. It could also give someone the power to spoil his enemy's deer hunting, to call the deer into the garden of an enemy, or to cause a particular disease in someone else.

After an encounter with a spirit, some reminder of the vision was kept in a special bag or pouch usually made from an animal skin. This was the famous medicine pouch, which contained the sacred religious objects of its owner—his pipe and tobacco, a

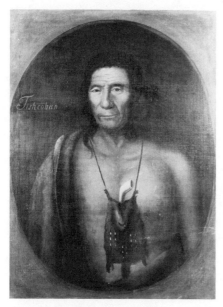

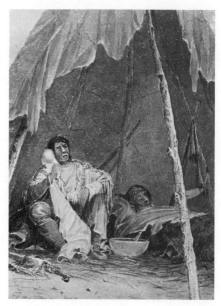

Around his neck this Delaware chief wears a beaded medicine pouch containing his pipe and other objects of religious significance.

A shaman, or medicine man, chants to the accompaniment of a rattling gourd in a ritual designed to heal a man stricken with disease.

stone, feather, hoof, claw, tail, or any item with special significance as a charm or memento. An Indian might have several encounters with a spirit in his lifetime, and each one added another power to his medicine bag. If he never had a vision at all, he might be able to buy some medicine from someone else who had more than enough. A man with special gifts, one to whom the spirits often spoke and whose charms had great success, especially in healing, might become a *shaman*, or medicine man.

In some tribes the shamans became persons of considerable power and wealth; in others the shaman was indistinguishable from his fellow tribesmen until he was called upon to perform his healing arts. It was assumed, however, that anyone who could cure disease could also cause it, and so shamans might be feared, hated, and accused of witchcraft.

American Indians believed that in order for man to live, the forces of nature had to be renewed each year. If the spirits of nature were angry or offended in some way, they withdrew their life-giving gifts—corn, rain, buffalo, salmon. Every man had two duties to perform so that he and his people might survive. He had to please the spirits by showing respect and gratitude, and he had to avoid offending or injuring them. Some tribes had great collective ceremonies that were held to insure the good luck of the tribe and the goodwill of the forces that ruled them. Ceremonies of the first fruit or the first game of the season were common. Tribal ceremonies such as the Buffalo Dance of the Mandans and the Green Corn ceremonies of many eastern tribes were intended to give thanks for the buffalo and the corn and to insure their abundance in the future.

All Indian societies were much concerned with disease and its cure. Indians used herbs, diet, and sweating in treating disease, but the magical part of the treatment was considered the most effective. Medicine societies conducted ceremonies to insure the health of the whole tribe. They might also try to cure individuals. Any individual who was known to have a special power to cure a particular disease, say snake-bite or tooth-ache, could be asked to help if his medicine was needed.

Dancing, singing, the use of tobacco, and acts of purification (fasting, bathing, sweating) were used everywhere among Indians as part of religious ceremonies. The great events of the human life cycle had religious importance. Special rites were observed at birth, puberty (especially of girls), and death. The Indians' profound reverence and respect for the living world and their belief in dreams and visions as spiritual experiences remain today as part of the legacy of Pre-Columbian Indian religion.

Social Behavior

Although Indians were often stereotyped as silent, stony-faced, dour people, this is a totally inaccurate picture. It is true that Indians were silent in situations of stress or anxiety. The ideal of bravery in many tribes was to bear pain without crying out. Silence was also used to show disapproval or social rejection. But laughter, games, and play were part of Indian life everywhere. Contests of skill and prowess—shooting, racing, wrestling—were favorites. Gambling games were played by both sexes. Many kinds of ball games were invented in North America, including the famous lacrosse of the northern tribes. Another ball game imported from Mexico was played in a large permanent court with a solid rubber ball. Teasing, joking, and trick playing were part of the Indians' daily life. Some societies even had rules regulating what kind of teasing was permissible between certain relatives. Myths of great supernatural tricksters, especially the Raven and the Coyote, were beloved by many tribes.

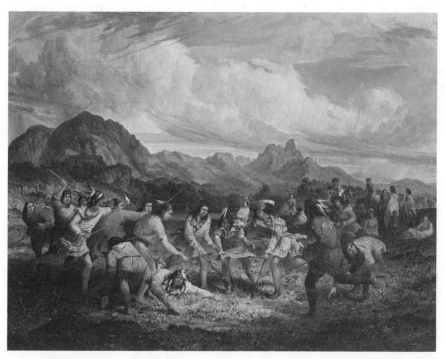

This picture by artist Seth Eastman captures the excitement and the highly competitive spirit of the Indian ball game lacrosse.

Population

Population varied in Pre-Columbian America according to food supply. In Mexico, intensive agriculture supported the largest population on the continent. But farming north of the Rio Grande was really gardening in most areas. Irrigation was practiced in Mexico and in the Southwest. Otherwise crops were raised in the simplest possible way. The universal farm tools were the wooden digging stick with a fire-hardened point and the hoe made of the shoulder blade of a deer or buffalo. Without the use of metal tools or animal power, Indian farmers had to keep their fields fairly small. Whenever possible, they were located on soil that was easy to cultivate, such as that on riverbanks or in natural clearings. Only a few groups on the Atlantic coast seem to have used fertilizer. Other Indians moved their fields as the fertility of the soil declined. The major improvement made in agriculture by the American Indians was the development of new varieties of corn that would survive and produce under the most difficult conditions.

Other factors influenced population throughout the continent. All Indians, whether they raised corn or not, depended on the bounty of nature for necessary food supplements—game, fish, and wild plants. Except on the Northwest and California coasts, want was an effective population control everywhere north of Mexico. Disease also limited population severely. It is estimated that only half the children in precontact America survived the age of five. Hunting was a hazardous occupation, and accidents carried off a large proportion of adult men. War also acted as a population control in those areas where it was part of the culture. In general there was a shortage of men.

Most tribes also had several ways of regulating their own numbers. Marriage was forbidden within the kin group. Birth control was built into religious and social customs. The most common regulation was to forbid sexual intercourse to nursing mothers. Since children were generally nursed until they were at least two, this rule provided for spacing of children. Sexual activity was limited in other ways. Men had to abstain often as a ritual preparation for the hunt, for war, or for some religious ceremony. Among some California Indians, men slept apart from women in a sort of men's club house except for certain periods of the year. Pre-Columbian Indians also had many methods of producing abortion. Such methods of birth control, combined with the effects of disease and want, limited the growth of Indian population. Authorities cannot agree in their estimate of population before Columbus, but the figure was probably under 1,000,000 for the area north of Mexico.

Arts and Crafts

No matter how difficult the conditions of their lives, the Indians of North America produced many objects of such fine design and excellent craftsmanship that they are truly works of art. The arts of American Indians are a most impressive contribution to the culture of mankind. Nomadic tribes applied most of their artistic efforts to necessary or useful items. Sedentary people were more free to make objects of primarily artistic importance. There was no art for art's sake, however. Even the great totem poles, the most elaborately carved masks, and the

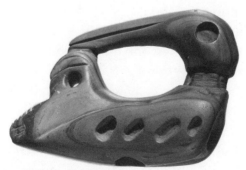

This gracefully designed stone pipe bowl was carved by an Indian craftsman of the Eastern Woodlands.

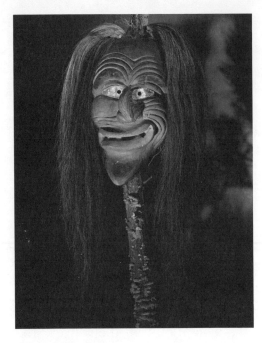

The Iroquois Indians used dramatic false-face masks such as this one to drive away evil spirits and disease.

grandest costumes had some social or religious purpose in addition to their artistic merit. A great variety of crafts—woodcarving, potting, basketmaking, embroidery, stone carving—and an exciting and vigorous design tradition are part of the American Indians' response to their environment.

It may seem from this incomplete list of shared traits that American Indian cultures had a great deal in common. To the native people, however, the differences among them were of far more importance than the similarities. Many tribes called themselves by names that mean "the human beings," or "the people," or just "the men." The tendency was to treat outsiders with suspicion, contempt, fear, or hate. There were many exceptions to this general attitude, and the trend since the appearance of the white man has been toward Indian unity. But disunity based on intertribal distrust was an important factor in the white conquest of the United States and has often worked against the best interests of all Indians.

PART II

Subsistence Areas

Beyond the culture traits that can be considered Amerindian lies a bewildering variety of tribal differences. In order to sort Indian tribes into more manageable categories, anthropologists have divided the continent into a number of geographical areas according to the major food resource of each one. In these *subsistence areas* tribes are grouped by their location and by their mode of subsistence before contact with white men changed their traditional way of life.

1. *The Arctic*

North of the line where trees stop is a region of barren, inhospitable tundra known as the Arctic. The same line divides a unique group of native Americans, the Eskimos, from the Indians of the Subarctic Woodlands. Men have been living in the Arctic as long as they have been on the continent, so that by 1000 B.C., when the immediate ancestors of the modern Eskimos arrived, they found a people who had already developed much that we think of as Eskimo culture.

The Eskimos themselves are late-comers to North America, and their racial characteristics are somewhat different from those of American Indians. Eskimos are short and stocky, and have a special layer of fat under the skin. They have the high cheek bones, flat face, and eye fold that are characteristic of Mongoloid people. There are local differences among the Eskimos of various

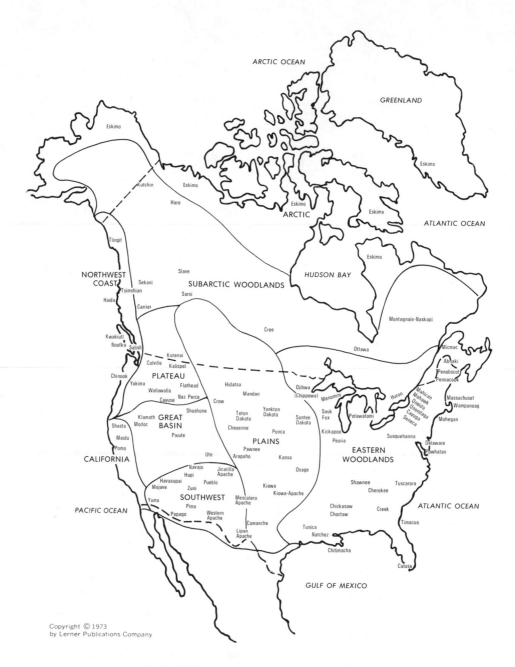

ARCTIC OCEAN

GREENLAND

Eskimo

Eskimo

Kutchin

Eskimo

Hare

Eskimo

ARCTIC

Eskimo

ATLANTIC OCEAN

Tlingit

NORTHWEST
COAST

Sekani

Slave

SUBARCTIC WOODLANDS

HUDSON BAY

Eskimo

Tsimshian

Sarsi

Montagnais-Naskapi

Haida

Carrier

Cree

Kwakiutl
Nootka

Salish

Ottawa

Micmac

Kutenai

Abnaki

Colville

Kalispel

Penobscot
Pennacook

Chinook

PLATEAU

Hidatsa

Ojibwa
(Chippewa)

Huron

Mahican
Mohawk

Massachuset

Yakima

Menomini

Oneida
Onondaga

Wampanoag

Wallawalla

Flathead

Mandan

Nez Perce

Cayuse

Crow

Potawatomi

Cayuga
Seneca

Shoshone

Teton
Dakota

Yankton
Dakota

Sauk
Fox

Mohegan

Klamath

GREAT
BASIN

Santee
Dakota

Shasta

Modoc

Cheyenne

Ponca

Kickapoo

Susquehanna

Maidu

Paiute

PLAINS

Peoria

EASTERN
WOODLANDS

Delaware

Pomo

Pawnee

Powhatan

CALIFORNIA

Ute

Arapaho

Kansa

Navajo

Jicarilla
Apache

Osage

Hopi

Havasupai

Pueblo

Kiowa

Shawnee

Cherokee

Tuscarora

Mojave

Zuni

Kiowa-Apache

Yuma

SOUTHWEST

Mescalero
Apache

Pima

ATLANTIC OCEAN

PACIFIC OCEAN

Papago

Western
Apache

Comanche

Chickasaw

Creek

Timacua

Lipan
Apache

Choctaw

Tunica

Natchez

Chitimacha

Calusa

GULF OF MEXICO

SUBSISTENCE AREAS AND TRIBAL LOCATIONS

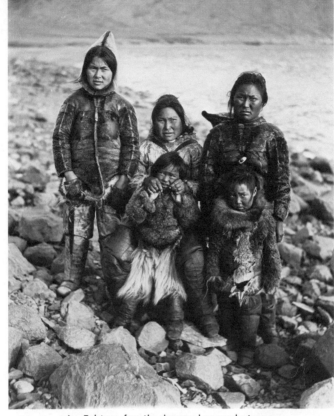

An Eskimo family dressed warmly in garments made of sealskin and caribou hide

regions, but there are no tribal differences as there are among Indians, and many culture traits, including language, are common to all.

In prehistoric times Eskimos were exclusively hunters. The Arctic Ocean provided the major element in their subsistence, the sea mammals—whale, walrus, and seal. Although there were a number of plant foods available to them, they ignored them in favor of animal foods. Because they ate much of their meat raw and because they ate all parts of the animal, including large proportions of fat, the Eskimo diet had all the elements necessary for good health when enough game was available. They also supplemented their diet with caribou, waterfowl, and fish taken inland during the brief summertime. (Eskimos developed many highly specialized tools for taking these animals.) Several families united to hunt the whale and walrus, but, except for these cooperative hunts, each Eskimo family was a self-contained survival unit.

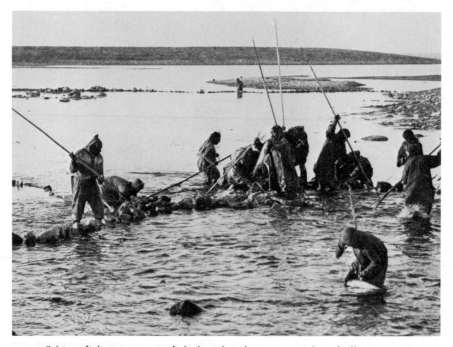

Eskimo fishermen spear fish that they have trapped in shallow water.

Eskimos were thinly scattered all round the polar region of North America. The Bering Strait Eskimo lived in the west, and the Copper, the Caribou, the Labrador, and the Greenland Eskimo in the east. The Polar Eskimos ranged as far north as the 79th degree of latitude; they were called the Raw Meat-Eaters by their Algonquin neighbors to the south.

The Eskimos have probably never numbered more than 50,000 to 70,000. Their highly specialized culture allowed them to live in one of the world's most forbidding climates. The struggle to sustain life in the Arctic is endless. Consequently, the Eskimos' society was simple and undemanding of their time and effort.

2. *The Subarctic Woodlands*

South of the barren Arctic tundra begins the inland forest region of the Subarctic. The climate of the region is a severe one, with long, very cold winters and heavy snowfall. Summers are short and warm. Agriculture is not possible in this area because of the short growing season, but the region provides a great variety of plant and animal resources. Most important of these is the caribou, a new world reindeer. Moose, rabbits, and a variety of other woodland animals are important supplementary game.

The tribes of the western Subarctic spoke languages of the Athabaskan family, many of which are mutually intelligible. The Kutchin, Hare, Slave, Sarsi, Carrier, and Sekani were some of the western tribes. East of Hudson's Bay were tribes which spoke Algonquian languages: the Algonquins, Montagnais-Naskapi, Crees, and Ottawa, to name a few.

The Subarctic people had an inland hunting culture. However, they had neither the reliable game supply of the Eskimos nor their specialized methods of hunting. They were more likely to be hungry than the Eskimos or even to be starving. Small bands of several related families worked together at the tasks of hunting and gathering foods. They followed a seasonal round of local resources. In early winter they had a cooperative caribou drive, in mid-winter, they fished. In summer women gathered wild berries and other plant foods, and prepared them for storage. Men traveled in search of game—moose, musk oxen, and caribou. These activities were directed by a chief hunter who was known to be the most successful and skillful provider in the band. He had no authority over the band; he simply gave instructions which others willingly followed. Families were free to come and go from the band as they pleased. Each band ranged over a territory of its own, hunting and foraging. They would fight to keep others out if necessary.

The Subarctic tribes preserved a way of life more like that of the earliest American Indians than any other. Their culture was simple; possessions, art, even memories were kept to a minimum by people who had to move often and travel light. In areas where they had some contact with other cultures they added much to their own way of life. In the west, borrowings were made from the Northwest Coast people and the Eskimos, both of which had more elaborate cultures than the Athabaskans. In the east both Eskimos and the Algonquins of the Eastern Woodlands influenced them.

3. *The Northwest Coast*

If there is a land of milk and honey in North America, it is surely the Northwest Coast of the Pacific Ocean. This narrow strip of land, along with its offshore islands, is divided from the rest of the continent by the rugged mountains of the Cordillera. Countless streams and rivers, including the two great continental rivers, the Fraser and the Columbia, drain these mountains and flow into the sea. The climate is temperate, mild, and moist. Forests of giant coniferous trees cover the western slopes of the mountains. Located close together as they are, the resources of the forests, sea, rivers, and coastline are easily available to the inhabitants.

Most important of all these resources are the salmon that live in the sea but fight their way upstream into fresh water to spawn. Salmon was the staple food of the Northwest Coast Indians. There is also a superabundance of other plant and animal foods in the area—sea mammals (whale, sea otter, and seal), fish from the sea, shellfish from the shoreline, migratory waterfowl, game and fur-bearing animals from the mountains. The land is lush

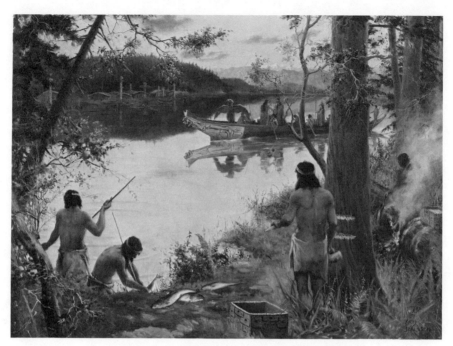

Indians of the Northwest Coast fish for salmon
in one of the teeming rivers of their homeland.

with vegetable foods of all kinds. Berries are especially abundant, and there is a great array of roots and greens.

Several language families are represented among the people of this region. Tribal names—Nootka, Chinook, Salish, Haida, Tsimshian, Tlingit—refer to language groups, not to tribal organizations. Northwest Coast society was organized around the house and the village. The houses were permanent buildings made of planks from the giant cedars that grew in nearby forests. In each house lived from six to ten nuclear families who were related through maternal lines. A house might have 60 inhabitants; a village, up to 12 houses. Everything about life in these villages differed sharply from the difficult existence of those Indians who lived in the far north.

The one aspect of the culture of the Northwest Coast tribes that most set them apart from other American natives was their attitude toward wealth. The natural abundance of their home-land made it possible to gather more than they could possibly use. Huge quantities of dried fish and other commodities were stockpiled in the great houses. This wealth was displayed at a public ceremony of feasting and gift-giving called a *potlach*. The easy abundance of life made possible not only the potlach but also many other social and religious ceremonies. Moreover, society on the Northwest Coast was organized in ranks according to wealth and inheritance. The material culture of the region was far richer than that of most other areas.

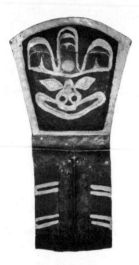

This painted copper shield, made by the Haida Indians of the Northwest Coast, was probably given as a gift at a potlach. The potlach was a public ceremony of feasting and gift-giving at which the Northwest Coast Indians displayed their great wealth.

In addition to the huge houses and boats that they built, the Northwest Coast tribes used their woodworking skill to fashion some outstanding contributions to native American art. The towering totem poles erected as symbolic family histories are a unique and unforgettable art form. Wooden storage boxes were decorated on all surfaces with design motifs that are unlike the decorations of any other Indian artisans. On a flat surface, an animal was represented as if it were split down the spine and flattened out to fill the space to be decorated. The result is not a naturalistic-looking animal but a dramatic abstract design. A few characteristics of each animal were always rendered in the same way so that it was clear which animal was being represented. A beaver, for instance, would have large incisor teeth, round ears, and a flat tail with cross-hatching. Some of the tribes of this area also wove wonderful blankets by a finger-weaving technique. The blankets were decorated with designs of the same kind that were used in woodcarving.

Though they raised no crops, made no pottery, and had no written language, the people of the Northwest Coast attained a cultural level more complex than that of any other nonagricultural society in the world. Their influence can be seen in the cultures of many peoples who lived around them.

4. *The American Desert*

With the exception of the coastal areas, the western part of the United States is arid country—the Great American Desert. This arid region lies between the Cordillera and the Rocky Mountains, extending from the Fraser River in British Columbia all the way to northern Mexico. From the Fraser to southeastern Oregon, the area is known as the Plateau. The land of the Plateau consists of wooded mountain slopes and flat sage desert. Great rivers drain the mountains; the river valleys are well watered.

South of the Plateau is the area known as the Great Basin. The mountains on either side block the basin's drainage to the sea and confine the waters from their slopes in marshes and lakes. The evaporation of these waters leaves behind alkaline and salt flats, marshes, and salt lakes such as the Great Salt Lake of Utah. The flatlands are hot, dry, and covered with various kinds of tough shrubbery such as sage and yucca. Sometimes they are completely barren salt and alkaline flats. The mountain slopes of the Basin are wooded and somewhat moister than the flatlands.

Most of California is similar to the Plateau and Basin. But in

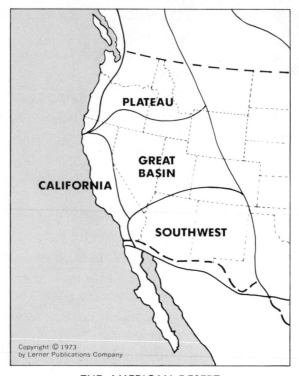

THE AMERICAN DESERT

addition to the arid and barren inland desert areas and the river valleys, there is also a coastal area rich in the resources of the sea: sea mammals, finny fish, and shellfish.

The Southwest—Arizona, New Mexico, western Texas, and Oklahoma—shares the desert landscape and climate. At its most severe the desert climate affects large parts of Nevada, Utah, eastern California, Arizona, and New Mexico. The Great Salt Desert in Utah has as little as five inches of rainfall per year. The entire state of Nevada has only a little over seven inches of rainfall per year. Of these vast desert areas, western California supplied the largest variety and most abundant food resources; the Great Basin, the least in both variety and quantity.

The mode of subsistence was similar for all desert dwellers. The staple of the desert diet was wild vegetable foods—nuts, seeds, roots, fruits, and berries. These foods were supplemented with hunting and fishing. In the Plateau the major food was roots; in the Basin, wild seeds; and in California, acorns. The one important exception to this mode of subsistence was in the Southwest. Here desert dwellers had added agriculture to their gathering life.

Like the tribes of the far north, the people of the desert were fully occupied with the food quest, except where agriculture was practiced. Their culture was simpler as a result. The wandering existence meant smaller, less organized groups, fewer possessions, and fewer and less elaborate religious and social customs.

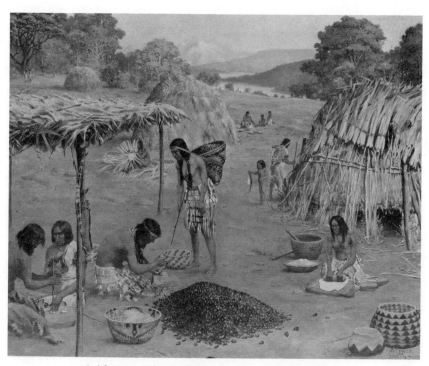

California Indians grind acorns into meal. Acorns provided the staple food for these desert dwellers.

The Plateau and the Basin

The Plateau was the home of many tribes speaking languages of several different families. Some well-known Plateau tribes were the Kutenais, Kalispels, Flatheads, Colvilles, Spokanes, Coeur d'Alenes, Wallawallas, Nez Perces, Yakimas, Cayuses, Klamaths, and Modocs. Generally these people lived in small, permanent winter villages located at sites along the rivers. Three to five extended families (30-40 persons) made up the average population of a village. Winter homes were round pit houses that accommodated several families.

During the spawning season, a year's supply of salmon and trout was caught, dried, and stored at the villages. Early in spring, families began to move out onto the desert to dig roots and tubers. These were also dried and stored. Later in the season, the people would move up the slopes to gather berries, and in the fall, men went to the mountains for game. The severest part of the winter was spent in the villages.

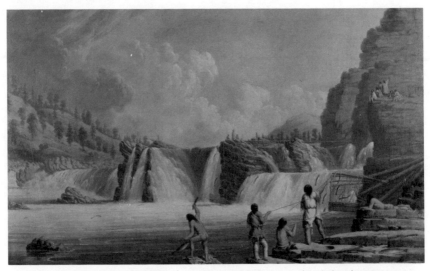

Indians of the Plateau fish for salmon at a falls on the Columbia River. The Indians use spears and basket traps to catch the salmon as they fight their way upstream during the spawning season.

Basin people spoke languages belonging to the Shoshonean branch of the Uto-Aztecan family. These people always seem to have been desert dwellers. The mighty Aztecs themselves, whose language belonged to this family, were probably wandering desert gatherers from the north when they came upon the rich cultures of central Mexico and settled down to become farmers and conquerors. But, except for the related languages, there is very little in the Basin way of life that suggests the complex and brilliant culture of the Aztecs. The Shoshone tribes of the Basin were scattered over widely differing territory, but their languages were mutually intelligible and they considered themselves related.

The Basin is drier, harsher, and more barren than the Plateau. Because there was no large or reliable supply of any one food, Basin people made use of practically every edible resource, including insects and reptiles. They searched for food in small bands, sometimes consisting of only one extended family—grandparents, parents, and children. Beginning on the flatlands in spring, the people of the Basin would gather green shoots and hunt antelope if any were available. In summer they would move up the slopes to dig roots, gather berries, and fish, especially for salmon. In the fall large crops of nuts (piñon and acorns) and seeds were gathered on the higher slopes. Rabbit and other game were available from time to time. An experienced elder directed the work of the hunting band. Occasionally several bands would unite in a temporary village to take advantage of some unusually large supply of food—rabbits or piñon nuts perhaps. When the food had been used, the bands went their separate ways.

Before the coming of the horse, war played little part in the lives of desert people. The highest ideal of most Plateau tribes was to live together in peace and harmony. The main responsibility of the village chief was to promote peace in every way possible, both within the village and between villages. Basin

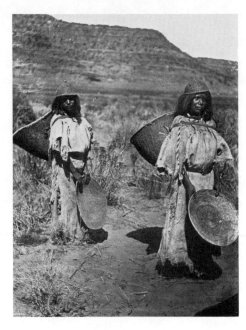

Women of the Paiute tribe on a seed-gathering expedition. Like all Basin people, the Paiutes spent most of their time searching for food.

people, who were called "Diggers" by the first white men who saw them, were timid and peaceable, and had time for little more than working for survival.

Horses came to the Basin from the Southwest and the Plains. Sometime after 1700, they reached the Plateau. For those whose lands would support them, horses brought a more abundant way of life. Buffalo hunting, tipis, skin clothing, and plains-style warfare were adopted along with horses. The Shoshone of Wyoming and Idaho were able to raise large herds of horses on their grassy lands. When the buffalo were all gone from their own country, they rode their horses far out onto the Plains for annual hunts. They also included fishing expeditions to the Plateau in their travels. Some Plateau tribes, notably the Nez Perces, Cayuses, and Yakimas, who lived on lands rich in grasses, became famous as horse herders and breeders. The much admired Apaloosa horses were developed by Plateau people. By the time white men met these Indians, they were following a way of life quite like that of the Plains people.

54

The Southwest

Sometime between 100 B.C. and 400 A.D., desert dwellers of the Southwest added agriculture to their hunting and gathering life. Farming and contacts with the cultures of Mexico set the stage for the highly developed Pueblo cultures. Though they continued to gather wild seeds and fruits and to hunt, corn culture became the central activity of their lives. They also raised beans, tobacco, and cotton in precontact times.

When the Spanish explorer Francisco Coronado arrived in the Southwest in 1540, he found 80 or more *pueblos*, or villages. Today 30 remain. Archaeologists study the cultures of these surviving pueblos in order to understand and interpret the remains of the pueblos now in ruins.

The 30 surviving pueblos are divided into two groups. The

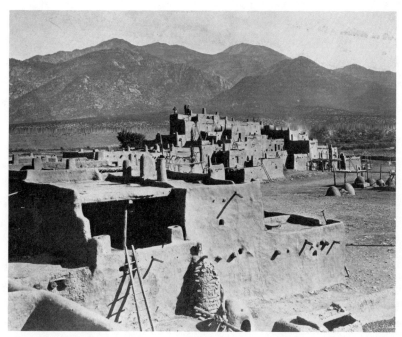

The Taos pueblo in New Mexico. Today, this terraced adobe village is occupied by Pueblo Indians whose ancestors lived in the Southwest centuries ago.

eastern villages are located along the Rio Grande in New Mexico. Five of them speak Keresan languages, the others speak languages belonging to the Tanoan family. These people locate their fields in river bottoms and irrigate them. The western Pueblos live in western New Mexico. They include the Zuñi, whose language is unrelated to any other, 12 Hopi villages whose languages belong to the Uto-Aztecan family, and two other Keresan-speaking villages, Acoma and Laguna. The western Pueblos engage in dry farming.

Other agricultural desert tribes that do not live in pueblos are the Pimas and Papagos of southern Arizona. In the west, along the Colorado River, live the Mojaves, Yumas, Yavapai, Walapai, Havasupai, and others less devoted to agriculture.

The terraced, many-storied stone and adobe apartment villages called pueblos (towns) by the Spanish were built on sites that offered a good defensive position somewhere near the fields and gardens. Groups of these buildings were arranged around a plaza where religious ceremonies were held. Somewhere within every pueblo were sacred chambers called *kivas*, where secret religious ceremonies took place.

The apartment-house style of architecture that developed among the Pueblos was symbolic of their coordinated, orderly, cooperative society, which was fully integrated into its environment. The object of life was for all members of the group to live harmoniously with each other and with the universe. Only if order and peace prevailed and the spirits of the dead were content would the rain fall, the harvest be good, and people and animals be healthy and fertile.

In addition to living quietly, industriously, and inconspicuously with their fellow men, the people of the pueblos tried to assure the harmony of the universe by a cycle of religious ceremonies observed throughout the year. Secret religious societies were responsible for the round of observances. The priests of the

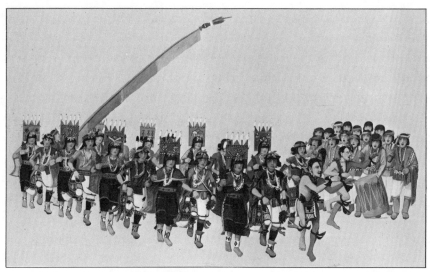

A modern Indian artist, **Fred Kabotie**, depicts the Hopi Corn Dance, an ancient ritual held to insure the fertility of the corn crop.

societies, who formed the town council, saw to it that the religious ceremonies took place on time. Members of the council also decided town policy and sat in judgment on anyone accused of a crime. A warrior society carried out the orders of the council and provided for defense.

In addition to the farming peoples, the Southwest was the home of several groups of nomadic Athabaskan-speaking people who came there from the north. The Athabaskans who inhabit the western Subarctic forests were nomadic hunters. Exactly when their nomadic relatives reached the Southwest is uncertain, but they were surely there by 1500 A.D., perhaps as early as 900 A.D. What is clear is that at the end of the 13th century the Pueblos began to wall up the doorways and gates to their towns and to take other defensive measures. During the same period, some of the northern pueblos were abandoned, leaving behind such evidence of violence as unburied and mutilated skeletons. Other pueblos were enlarged at this time, possibly by refugees.

The trees used for beams in the construction of the pueblos show that there was a long, severe drought between the years 1276 and 1299. Perhaps newly arrived Athabaskans were making war on the settled population during these years. Perhaps famine, which surely accompanied the drought, forced them to raid the pueblos for food. These nomadic invaders were the ancestors of the Navajos and several groups of Apaches—Jicarilla, Chiricahua, Lipan, and Kiowas.

The Navajos and Apaches went on with their hunting and gathering life in their new home. Gradually they borrowed some of the ways of their settled neighbors. When the Pueblos acquired horses and other livestock from the Spanish, the Apaches and Navajos soon helped themselves to their neighbors' animals. The Apaches were foot people, and they did not become horse breeders. They used horses for raiding both white and Pueblo settlements. Then they traded the horses with tribes to the north. But the horse was never integrated into the Apache way of life. When a horse was no longer useful to an Apache, he was willing to sell it, trade it, or eat it, whichever was most practical. Navajos also carried on raids against their neighbors, but, in addition to trading the stock, they became herders and breeders of sheep and horses. The Navajos changed most in the Southwest, developing a distinctive culture made up of elements acquired from both the Pueblos and the whites, and from their Athabaskan past.

The peoples of the Southwest created many well-known and highly regarded objects of art. Their design traditions go far back into prehistoric times. Pueblo pottery was made by women using the coiling method (in this method of pottery making, ropes of wet clay are coiled one on top of another on a clay base). The pottery was then painted with beautiful designs, usually geometric in character. Highly prized pottery is still being made in a few of the pueblos.

Southwestern textiles are also extraordinary. In the pueblos men did the weaving; they produced cotton cloth in a wide variety of weaves and designs. After white men introduced sheep and the rigid loom, Navajo women took up the craft. The rugs and blankets they produced are important artistic creations. Jewelry of silver set with turquoise and other semiprecious materials was also made by the Navajos and the Zuñi. The technique of metal working was introduced by white men, but the jewelry is native in both design and character. Katchina dolls, masks and costumes for religious ceremonies, and sand paintings made for ritual purposes all qualify as arresting works of art.

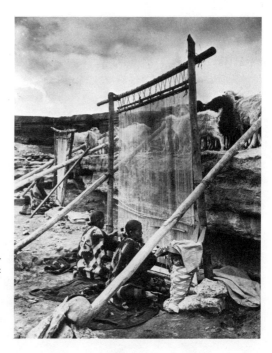

Navajo women practice their tribe's ancient tradition of weaving.

The basketry of the desert people was skillfully and artistically made to serve many different purposes. Depending on the tribe and the locality, hats, fish traps, and baby cradles were fashioned from basketry. Bowls, trays, and water jugs (smeared with pitch to make them waterproof), gathering and storage baskets, water-tight baskets for stone boiling were all manufactured from plant materials. These articles were often beautifully ornamented with woven or embroidered designs similar to those used on pottery.

5. *The Eastern Woodlands*

The area between the Atlantic Ocean and the Mississippi River, from the St. Lawrence River in the north to the Gulf of Mexico in the south, is known as the Eastern Woodlands. Its wooded hills and valleys are well watered by a network of streams, rivers, and lakes. The features of the land tend to divide it into separate subsistence pockets. In the north the area of effective agriculture ends north of the Great Lakes; the prairies begin west of the Mississippi.

In the northern area the majority of tribes belonged to the Algonquian language family. Many tribal names recall colonial history and remain as place names to the present. In Nova Scotia and New Brunswick lived the Micmacs and Malacites; in Maine,

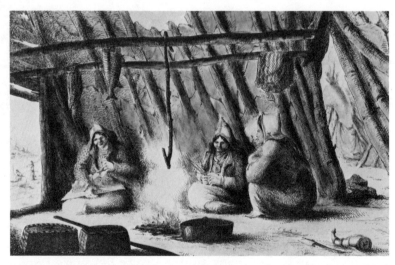

Interior of a Micmac lodge. The Micmacs, who lived in the Northeast Woodlands, were primarily hunters and fishermen.

the Penobscots and the Abnaki; in New England, the Pennacooks, Massachusetts, Wampanoags, Pequots, Narragansetts, Mohegans, and Mahicans, and farther to the south, the Delawares. The Conestogas and Susquehannas lived farther inland.

In the Middle West (Ohio, Illinois, Michigan, Indiana) were the Potawatomies, Sauk and Fox, Menominis, Kickapoos, Kaskaskias, and Peorias. North of the Great Lakes were Chippewas, Ottawas, and Algonquins. Surrounded on all sides by these Algonquin-speaking tribes were several Iroquoian groups: the Seneca, Mohawk, Oneida, Onondaga, Cayuga, Erie, and Huron tribes. They lived around the upper Great Lakes in New York State and Pennsylvania. At the time of contact, several Siouan-speaking tribes also lived in the Eastern Woodlands—the Winnebagos of Wisconsin-Michigan and several groups of Dakota (Sioux) in Minnesota and western Wisconsin.

Woodland culture was basic to over half the area that is now the United States, and much that we think of as "Indian" culture originates in the Woodland way of life. The foundation of subsistence in the Woodlands was corn culture, but dependence on agriculture varied across this vast area. Supplements to food supplied by farming, especially game, were very important everywhere.

The Algonquins of the Northeast were generally less devoted to agriculture than the neighboring Iroquois, and their social and political organization was not so elaborate. In the central part of the Northeast Woodlands, summer villages with nearby fields were located in choice agricultural spots along the rivers. These villages were usually occupied during the growing season, but they were deserted during the winter when the people separated into smaller bands. Farther north agriculture could provide only a minor part of subsistence. In this area tribes such as the Abnaki, Penobscot, Ottawa, and Chippewa followed the seasonal development of food resources, moving from sugar camps, to fish camps, to garden villages, to hunting camps.

The major game animal of the Woodlands was the Virginia, or white-tailed, deer. Lakes and streams provided fish almost everywhere. (Fish were a major item in the diet of the Huron and the Chippewa.) Wild rice, which grows along the marshy shores of lakes, was harvested as a staple grain by the Indians of the Minnesota-Wisconsin lakes region.

Clothing worn by the Indians of the Eastern Woodlands was made of deerskin and fur. Birchbark folded and stitched into shape was used to make all kinds of containers—trays, baskets, buckets. Some pottery was made, and other utensils were carved of wood. Homes were round or oval pole structures, usually dome-shaped (the wigwam) and covered with mats or bark.

The Algonquins of the Eastern Woodlands and their Subarctic neighbors used snowshoes to pursue game and travel in the winter woods. These "big feet" allowed a man to move along on the surface of deep snow without breaking through. For summer transport and travel the Northeastern tribes developed a near perfect vehicle—the birchbark canoe. It was light, strong, and

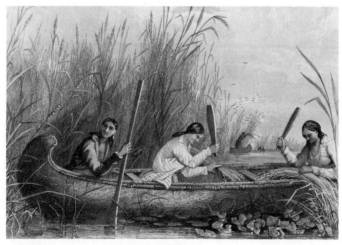

Chippewa women harvesting wild rice, a staple grain in some areas of the Eastern Woodlands

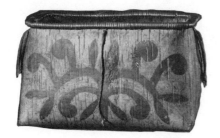
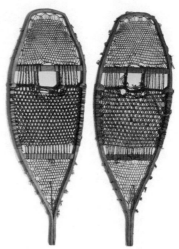

This birchbark container and pair of snowshoes are typical of the beautiful and functional products made by the craftsmen of the Eastern Woodlands.

maneuverable, and it could easily be carried where water was impassable. The forests supplied cedar for the framework of the canoe, birchbark to cover it, spruce roots for stitching, and pitch to caulk the seams.

Iroquois society, though based on the same general way of life, was elaborated beyond that of other Northeastern tribes. The Iroquois were more populous, led a more sedentary life, and depended more upon agriculture than their Algonquin neighbors did. Iroquois agriculture supported large fortified towns. Community ceremonial life among the Iroquois was rich and complex. Their celebrations, which followed the agricultural cycle, were held to insure fertility and to give thanks. The Green Corn Festival was the most important of these celebrations.

The Iroquois were able to dominate the northern lakes region because they had developed an inter-tribal alliance. This famous alliance—the Iroquois League—united five Iroquois tribes of upper New York State. Although the original intention of the alliance was to keep peace among these tribes, the final effect was to give the League the balance of power in warfare. The

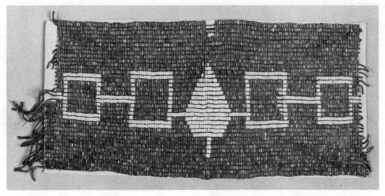

The symbols on this wampum belt represent the five tribes making up the Iroquois League. The symbol in the center stands for the Onondaga tribe, which had the largest number of representatives on the League council.

League council, which made the League decisions, was originally made up of 50 *sachems*, or tribal leaders: 14 Onondaga, 9 Mohawk, 10 Cayuga, 9 Seneca, and 8 Oneida. These positions on the council were inherited by men through their mothers; great prestige and influence went with them. The League council did not interfere in internal tribal affairs, but the sachems were also members of tribal councils. Such large and powerful Iroquois groups as the Hurons and Eries were not part of the League and were often at war with it.

In the milder climates of the Southeast Woodlands, agriculture sustained larger populations than were common in the north. The Indians of the Southeast tended to be more sedentary and more highly organized. Many of them, especially those who lived along the Gulf and the lower Mississippi, inherited much from the highly developed mound-building cultures that preceded them.

A few of the most familiar tribes of the Southeast Woodlands were the Algonquin Powhatans of the Virginia coast, and the inland Shawnees. The Tuscaroras of the Carolina coast and the Cherokees of the hills inland were Iroquoian-speaking people. Representatives of several other unrelated language families such as the Natchez, Tunica, and Chitamacha lived along the lower Mississippi and the Gulf Coast. The largest group was made up of the Muskogean-speaking tribes: the Creeks, Chickasaws, Choctows, Timacuas, and Calusas. The Creeks and the Cherokees were the largest tribes in the Southeast at the time of contact with the white man.

The southeastern Indians lived in villages and towns located near streams and rivers. Each town had a chief. A few tribes, notably the Natchez and the Powhatans, had a supreme chief who ruled over the whole tribe. Early European observers were likely to refer to these tribal heads as "kings," and, in fact, they did have more in common with old-world kings than any other chieftains north of Mexico.

Such "kings" usually inherited their positions, and their relatives were treated as a noble class. Their public duties included

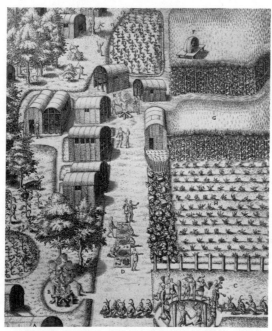

A 16th-century drawing of an Indian village in the Southeast Woodlands. The village's carefully cultivated fields of tobacco, corn, and other vegetables indicate the high level of subsistence in this area.

presiding over the yearly round of religious ceremonies, maintaining the community fields and storehouses, and overseeing large-scale war activities. The chiefs had finer, larger houses, more food, and more wives than ordinary people. They were treated with great deference and respect, and they had absolute authority, including life and death power. Such absolute authority was the exception rather than the rule among North American Indians. This kind of political organization and the religious ideas that were associated with it seem to have originated in Mexico.

For most southeastern people, such as the Creeks, Cherokees, Choctows, and Chickasaws, life was somewhat simpler. These tribes cultivated community fields as well as family gardens. Men shared in the agricultural work in the community fields, and the chiefs of the villages had the power to force shirkers to do their share. The produce from the community fields went into community storehouses to be used in times of emergency and war. Family gardens were generally tended by women, except for the heavy work of clearing and harvesting. Men spent about half their time hunting.

Throughout the Woodlands, men were thought of primarily as warriors, and their social standing was based on their prowess in war. A victory meant prestige for the winning tribe, as well as personal glory for individual warriors. Trophies of some kind, usually scalps, were taken as proof of success. Personal ambition played a part in the decision to make war, especially for untried young men, but revenge was usually the official reason given. The community might decide to pay back an earlier raid, or a warrior might organize a war party to avenge the death of a relative.

In Pre-Columbian times loot was not a factor in a decision to make war. Conquered villages with all their stores were usually burned. Moreover, acquiring territory was never the object of war. Captured women and children were enslaved, though most of them eventually married into the tribe. Young warriors might also be spared, but a veteran warrior with many trophies or tattoos was certain to be tortured to death by the victorious villagers in a public ceremony.

The rules of war among the Woodland Indians were totally unlike those of Europeans. There were traditional enemies among the tribes, but there were no sustained campaigns meant to end a war by winning it. Instead, most warring was done by small

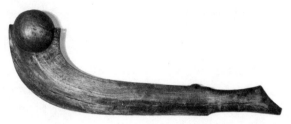

A wooden war club made by the Sauk and Fox tribe. Warfare was an important part of life among the Sauk and Fox and other Woodland Indians.

parties of willing volunteers whose attacks were made in a hit-and-run, guerilla style. A party might be organized when a war chief who had earned his title by his good war record announced his intention to go to war. There was no draft; only the willing joined the war party. The men followed their war chief out of respect for his ability, but if they thought the campaign was being badly managed, they were not obliged to follow his orders. He was a leader only, not a general. The war chief was responsible for the success of the venture, however. His strategy, therefore, was to get the maximum number of scalps with the minimum amount of injury to his own force. He would usually attack at dawn and quickly withdraw. He would never deliberately engage a larger force or stand and fight a losing battle if it were possible to retreat.

When the warriors returned with their trophies there was a

community celebration, usually a scalp dance or perhaps the execution of prisoners by torture and burning. Warriors might receive feathers, tattoos, and new titles as symbols of their success. War honors brought prestige and power to individual warriors, and eventually the high position of war chief.

The feelings of Woodland tribes toward war seem to be similar to those we are familiar with today. War was inescapable, a part of the social system. Because of it, society allowed periodic frenzies of blood and destruction, and associated glory and prestige with them. But Woodland people seemed to acknowledge that peace was really better than war. The confederations of the Creeks and Iroquois tribes were originally meant to end fighting between related groups. All tribes had some machinery for keeping and promoting peace. For many, the village chief was primarily a peace officer who tried to discourage war ventures. Although warfare was a well-developed part of the social system in the Eastern Woodlands, there is no doubt that people were of two minds about it.

The ceremonial life of the southeastern tribes tended to be more elaborate than that of the northern tribes, but it was based on the same ideas. Organized religious festivals involving the whole community followed the yearly growth cycle. The largest and most important was usually some kind of harvest festival. For the Creeks, this was the *Busk*, or Green Corn Festival.

The Busk was a ceremonial of both renewal and thanksgiving. It took place when the first of the new corn was in the roasting-ear stage. During the Busk all citizens purified themselves symbolically of their sins of the past year. They bathed and fasted, and the men took an emetic, the "black drink," which was prepared for them by priests. All crimes except murder were forgiven during the festival, and people came out of hiding to take part. Marriages that had taken place during the year became official after the Busk. Every household destroyed old clothes and tools, and began the year with new ones. At the end of the festival, the household fires were extinguished and relighted from the ceremonial fire in the town square. These rites and others, including dancing and feasting, were part of the four-day ceremonial. Other less elaborate feasts were held to celebrate the appearance of strawberries, deer, and other important foods.

6. *The Great Plains*

Across the entire center of the continent, from the Mississippi to the foothills of the Rockies, roll the seemingly endless grasslands of the Great Plains. From east to west the rainfall decreases so that the long lush grasses of the east gradually give way in the west to shorter, sparser grasses, cacti, and sagebrush. For the numberless herds of bison and antelope that once ranged in the

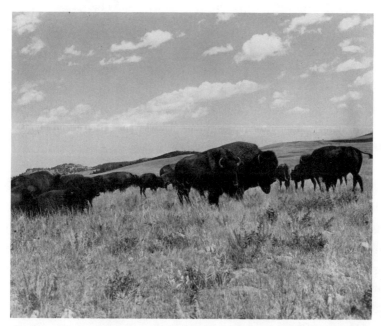

These buffalo grazing in a South Dakota state park are only a small remnant of the vast herds that once roamed over the Great Plains.

area, the plains were one enormous pasture. The region is drained by broad rivers that flow slowly through shallow channels and flat bottomlands. The rivers carry with them a heavy burden of silt that gives them a brown, gray, or yellow color. They are bordered by considerable stands of trees that provide a restricted woodland environment.

The rolling seas of grass were not a hospitable place for the prehistoric Indians who traveled on foot. Along the prairie rivers, however, they found water, a variety of woods for fires, lodges, and tools, and woodland plants and animals. The thick prairie sod would not yield to the simple hand tools of the women farmers, but the river bottomlands were easy to work. They were rich from deposits of silt, stayed moist longer in dry periods, and were protected from frost both early and late in the year.

In prehistoric times, farming people from the Eastern Woodlands moved out onto the Plains, following the river valleys. In the north Siouan-speaking people followed the drainage of the Missouri River. They were the ancestors of the historic Mandan, Hidatsa, Ponca, Osage, Iowa, Oto, Kansa, Omaha, and Missouri tribes. Farther south, Caddoan speakers followed the same pattern along the Kansas and Red rivers. These farming people from the Woodlands became the semisedentary Plains Indians who lived in permanent towns near their corn and went out on periodic hunts for buffalo, the other staple of their diet.

Eventually people of six different language families lived on the Plains. But only a few—the eastern Shoshone, Blackfoot, and Arapahoe-Gros Ventres in the north, and the Kiowa, Kiowa-Apaches, and Pawnee in the south—were certainly there in prehistoric times. The Shoshonean tribes—the Utes and Comanches—moved into the Plains from the Basin. The Kiowa-Apaches migrated from the Subarctic to the Southwest, and from there onto the Plains.

When horses reached the Plains, most tribes living there

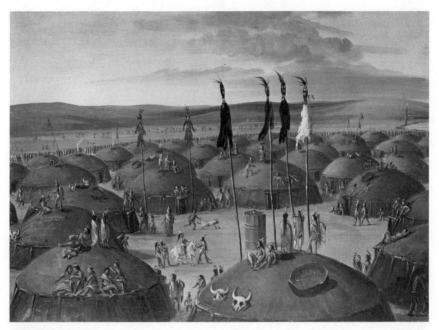

A bird's-eye view of a Mandan village, sketched by George Catlin. The Mandan Indians were farmers and hunters who lived in permanent villages located near their fields.

grafted the life of mounted buffalo hunting onto a foundation of Woodland culture. Some of the tribes that seem to be typical of the Plains buffalo hunters, such as the Sioux, Crow, and Cheyenne, actually found their way to the Plains in historic times. They gave up farming, pottery, and boats, and devoted themselves entirely to the nomadic way of life.

The nomadic hunting tribes of the Plains are probably the best known of the American Indians. This may be true partly because the Plains themselves, with their enormous herds of buffalo, were so impressive to the white men who first saw them. Early travelers speak of herds that blackened the prairie as far as the eye could see. Equally impressive were the people of the Plains, with their spectacular skill as horsemen, their daring and effective hunting methods, and their beautiful, dramatic costumes,

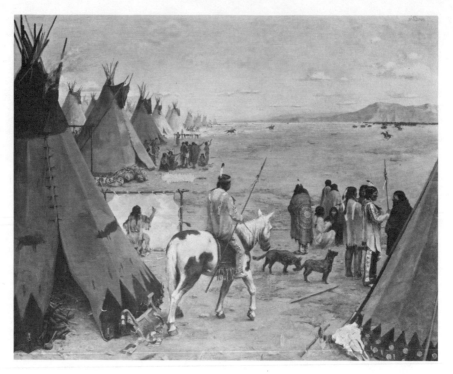

The tipis of the nomadic Plains tribes could be folded up and moved
from place to place as the Indians wandered in search of game.

including the familiar eagle feather war bonnet. The fame of
the Plains Indians is also due, no doubt, partly to the fact that
they were the last to give up their way of life and freedom, and
that they gave it up so reluctantly and at such great cost to the
white invaders.

It is ironic that the exciting Plains way of life that so impressed
the white men depended upon the horse, which was brought to
the Western Hemisphere *by* white men. When the Pueblo Indians
revolted in 1680, they acquired herds of Spanish horses. By 1740,
long before they ever saw a white man, Indians as far away as
Canada were using them. Horses were almost as much at home
on the Plains as the buffalo. Runaway horses went wild, and wild
herds provided another source of animals for those who could

capture them. Some of the southern tribes became horse-traders, raiding in the Southwest and in Mexico and trading and selling the animals to people from the north. The Indians did not have to be told what to do with horses. They seemed to be exactly what the Plains people had been waiting for. In a relatively short time, the horse became the standard of value among the Plains Indians, and a whole tradition of horsemanship developed.

With horses, buffalo hunting became more practical and efficient. The Plains Indians began to concentrate on the buffalo, neglecting other forms of subsistence. Father Nicholas Point, a Jesuit missionary to the Blackfeet, Coeur d'Alenes, and Flatheads in the 1840s, said that buffalo were to the Indians what manna in the desert was to the Israelites. The hump and tongue were considered the choicest parts of the fresh carcass. Most of the meat was "jerked" (cut in thin strips) and sun-dried on pole racks. Later it was pounded and mixed with dried, pounded berries or wild cherries, marrow, and melted fat to form *pemmican*, an easy-to-carry, dehydrated foodstuff of high nutritional value.

Preparation of the buffalo hides was a whole industry in itself. With the hair on, the hides became robes and bedding for cold weather. Clothing and all kinds of receptacles and containers were made from buffalo hide from which the hair had been removed. A characteristic Plains container, the *parfleche*, was a case for the storage of pemmican. It was made by folding a piece of hide into a large envelope and securing it with thongs. The Indians also used buffalo hide in making shelters. The Woodland tipi was elaborated into the grand Plains version, which sometimes had poles 40 feet long and needed from 14 to 18 buffalo skins for the covering.

Buffalo hide was also used to make tools and weapons. The stone mallet was an all-purpose tool used for driving stakes, breaking bones to extract marrow, dispatching wounded buffalo, pounding pemmican, and striking enemies. It was made by

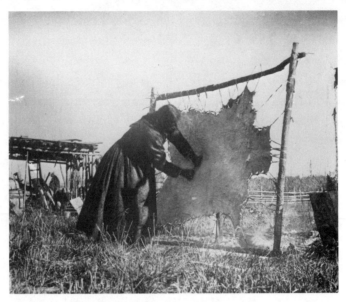
A Sioux woman prepares a buffalo hide stretched on a frame.

sewing the stone head into a piece of rawhide which was then attached to a handle. When the rawhide dried and stiffened, the stone head and the handle were pulled firmly together. Warriors made small round shields of buffalo rawhide that were so tough they could stop a rifle ball. Miles of cordage and "rope" needed for tying up bundles, tethering horses, and securing poles were cut from hide. Buffalo hooves were boiled to make the glue indispensable to the manufacture of a durable bow; buffalo sinew provided the bowstrings. Spoons were fashioned from horn, and some horns found their way into headdresses.

The methods of hunting buffalo with horses brought a more prosperous life to Plains people. Women were responsible for the buffalo carcass from the time the hunter brought it down. Thus they became increasingly valuable, and it became common for a man to have more than one wife. A great hunter who owned many horses and buffalo robes and was able to provide for several wives was a rich man. His wealth, however, only brought him prestige among his people if he gave it away freely to poor people, widows, and orphans, and used it to provide feasts and ceremonies for relatives and friends.

On the Plains, Woodland-style warfare was elaborated. The hit-and-run attack became a formidable war tactic when performed by mounted warriors. The system of trophies and honors was also elaborated. Honors were given not only for the taking of scalps but also for *coups*, or touches. A coup could be counted for any of several war exploits—killing an enemy, touching a live enemy in battle, touching an enemy corpse in battle, stealing a horse out of an enemy camp, or killing an enemy by stealth in his camp.

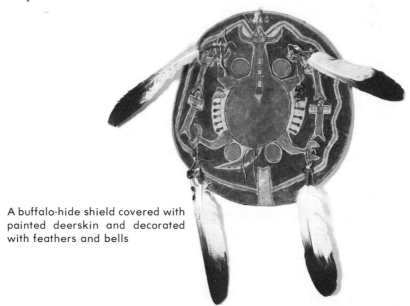

A buffalo-hide shield covered with painted deerskin and decorated with feathers and bells

Generous and protective toward their own people but fierce and implacable toward their enemies, the Plains Indians acquired the reputation of being the greatest of North American warriors. The ideal of a Plains warrior was to be brave, generous, enduring, and honest.

PART III

Red and White — The Colonial Period

1. *The Old World and the New: a Comparison*

By 1492, the tribes of western Europe had become "civilized." The people of Europe lived in a world very different from the world of the American Indian. In contrast to the loose, democratic political organization in most American tribes, Europeans lived in nation-states with highly centralized, authoritarian governments headed by hereditary kings. European society was organized in rigid classes. A small class of hereditary land owners, the aristocracy, held a very large share of the land, wealth, power, and prestige in both government and society. A large lower class of laborers worked for others and received a meager subsistence in return. For most of them, life held little more than grinding labor and poverty. In between these two classes was a small middle class engaged in buying, selling, and manufacturing in the cities. For the middle class, wealth could be the gateway to power and prestige, but most people expected to live just as their fathers had lived.

European cultural achievements of the 15th and 16th centuries were impressive. Great contributions were made in science, technology, art, architecture, philosophy, literature, and music. But, except for the land-owning class of nobles, the prosperous merchants, and the learned clergy of the church, most people were not much affected by the higher achievements of their culture.

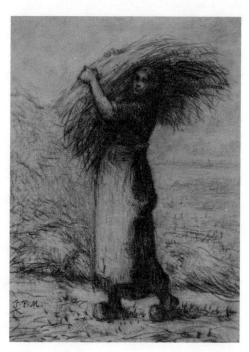

The life of the peasant in "civilized" Europe was traditionally one of poverty and hard work.

Europeans also shared a religion and a world view that were totally unlike those of the native Americans. Christianity took many forms, but some basic religious ideas were shared by all Christians. Implicit in all their activities was the attitude that man was the center of the universe. It was the *human* soul that God was interested in above all. Man, created in God's image, a little lower than the angels, was the measure of all things. The rest of creation was simply meant to sustain him and was his to subdue. The Europeans, as Christians, believed themselves to be the "chosen people," God's children. Non-Christians were heathens, pagans, devil-worshippers . . . in short, they were bad.

The age of crusading against the infidel Moslems was nearly over by the 15th century, but the crusading spirit was still strong. It was the mission of believers to rid the world of nonbelievers, either by converting them to the true faith or, failing that, by fire and sword. The church militant put far more emphasis on faith than it did on the Christian principles of love, peace, and brotherhood. At times disputes grew up among Christians over just what

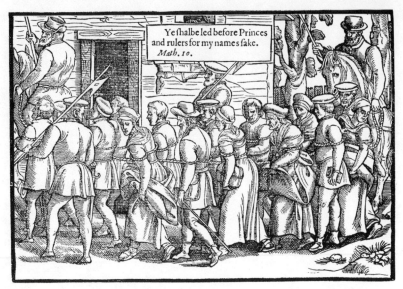

This drawing shows English Protestants being imprisoned because of their religion. Religious persecution such as this was a fact of life in Europe during the 15th and 16th centuries.

the "true faith" really was. Small groups of people broke away from the established church to follow their own version of Christianity. They were regularly denounced as heretics, persecuted, and executed. Strangely, their own experience as dissenters never seemed to make them more tolerant of other religious views.

Life was just as hazardous in Europe as it was in the New World. People were helpless against the famine, plague, and warfare that troubled them time and again. They were also at the mercy of the power of church and state. The usual fate of religious dissenters was to be burned alive. Political prisoners were tortured on ingenious machines and then beheaded. Dead bodies of traitors and dissenters were mutilated, cut up, skinned, and eviscerated, and their heads were hung on pikes. Ordinary criminals, from murderers to pick-pockets, were mutilated alive. Ears, noses, hands, and tongues were cut off. For minor crimes flogging and branding were typical punishments. There was nothing more "savage" in America.

2. *Colonization in the New World*

The power of European monarchs in the 15th century rested on successful military organizations. To consolidate, expand, and protect their power, generations of monarchs had been warring with each other. It was all very expensive. By the 15th century, royal treasuries were short of treasure.

There were other drains on the treasuries of the European nations during this period. The merchants of Europe needed gold and silver coin to buy the exotic products of the Far East from the middlemen of the Mediterranean. By the 15th century, important mines had run out. Other mines could not meet the demand, and so there was a shortage of precious metals for commerce. Any nation that could find a direct sea route to India and China would be able to avoid the gold-hungry Mediterranean traders, reduce the cost of transportation, and gain an advantage in world trade. The Portuguese, Dutch, Spanish, English, and French were all searching for such a route.

The Portuguese led the way around Africa, but that route was long and dangerous. Though his idea was not new, Columbus was the first man daring enough to try to reach the Far East by sailing west. When he did find land, he mistakenly believed that he had reached an island off the coast of India. So he made another mistake and called the native people he met there "Indians." Everyone soon knew that he had failed to find the new route to the east, but the name "Indians" remained. The confusion it causes has been a nuisance ever since. It was the first of many wrong judgments that white men made about native Americans.

Stories of the early voyages were soon circulating in Europe, and maps and descriptions of the new lands encouraged further efforts. Everyone expected that the coveted treasure mines would be found somewhere in the unexplored new world. Thus royal governments and wealthy people saw the explorations as a good

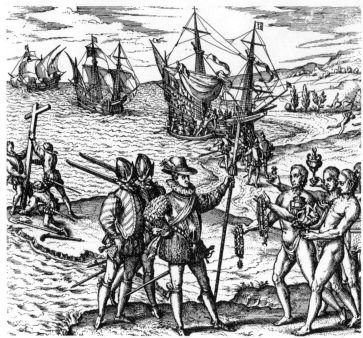
Columbus sought an overseas route to India but discovered instead the rich continent of America.

gamble. They financed voyages that they hoped would bring a good return on their investment. Governments assured themselves of a share in the discoveries by issuing official "permission slips" to explorers. Queen Elizabeth I, for instance, "gave" Sir Walter Raleigh any land he could find that was not inhabited by Christian people. All she asked in return was one-fifth of any gold and silver he might find on his property. Sir Francis Drake and others received similar grants and charters. Soon the seas were swarming with ships bearing the insignia and adventurers of England, Spain, France, Portugal, Holland, and other countries.

In 1492 Columbus landed in the West Indies. In 1513 Ponce de Leon discovered Florida. By 1565 there was a permanent settlement at St. Augustine, Florida. By 1521 Hernando Cortes had conquered the Aztecs in Mexico. In 1540 Spanish soldiers first entered the pueblos of New Mexico. By 1598 they were in the process of establishing permanent white settlements there.

Jacques Cartier, representing France, sailed up the St. Lawrence River as far as the present site of Montreal in 1535. By 1550 Frenchmen were regularly trading for furs with the Indians around the Gulf of St. Lawrence. By 1623 the French had explored as far west as Lake Superior. New France was a permanent, completely organized colony by 1635.

The English established their first permanent settlement in America at Jamestown in 1607. There was another settlement at Plymouth in 1620, and one at Charleston by 1669.

In 1769 the Spanish established a mission at San Diego, the first in California. English, American, and Russian ships began to trade with the Indians of the Northwest Coast after the visit of Captain James Cook to Vancouver Island in 1778. The assault on the continent came from all four quarters, and explorers from many European nations claimed lands and sovereignty for their kings.

Of all the greedy seekers, only the Spanish found treasure. Mexico and Peru gave up shipload after shipload of gold and silver. First the Spanish took the stockpiles of the Indians, and

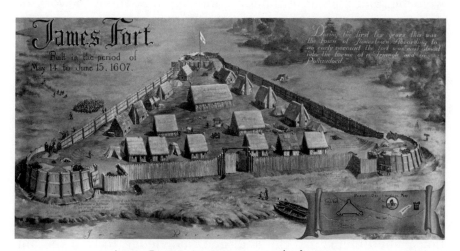

James Fort, or Jamestown, was the first permanent English settlement in North America.

later they mined more treasure, using forced Indian labor. Once the explorers realized that a whole new world lay between them and the Orient, they began to look for a waterway through it. But no one found the direct route to the east—the so-called "Northwest Passage" proved to be a will-o-the-wisp. So the disappointed treasure hunters turned their attention to extracting wealth from what they did find—the real treasure of the earth. The seas were full of fish, the forests full of timber, game, furs, and the lands rich with new and exotic crops.

Once the Spanish had secured the treasure of the Aztecs and the Incas, they moved north to Florida, New Mexico, and California, looking for more precious metals. When they found none, they established plantations instead. A group of Spanish adventurers received permission from the governor of Mexico to operate plantations, or *encomiendas*, in New Mexico. The Spanish encomienda system gave the plantation managers the "legal right" to use the forced labor of the native people. Instead of bringing large numbers of craftsmen from Spain, the Spanish taught the peaceful Pueblo Indians the skills of metal working, weaving, and animal husbandry, and required them to work on the plantations. The Indians received only a tiny share of what they produced. In Florida and California, the Catholic Church established missions to convert the Indians to Christianity and to teach them the "civilized arts." "Mission Indians" were compelled to work on the church lands and to practice the Catholic religion.

The French were probably most successful at getting the largest return for their investment in the New World. The rich furs of the northern animals were always a sought-after luxury in Europe. There was a steady demand for beaver pelts, which were used for hat making. Styles changed, but some kind of beaver hat was part of a European man's wardrobe for many generations. The Indians had the skill and knowledge to trap the animals, and the French gave them fairly inexpensive metal tools

82

and utensils, cloth, beads, and firearms in exchange for tons of animal pelts.

The French contribution to the fur trade was the trading organization that brought the furs out of the wilderness and back to the market. Trading posts far inland were served by the *voyageurs*, who brought the trade goods to the interior and returned to the St. Lawrence seaports with each season's catch. The enormous canoes the voyageurs used to navigate the Great Lakes were modeled after the much smaller birchbark craft used by the Indians.

The French, of all the Europeans, meddled least with the Indian way of life, although competition for furs soon brought the Indians into conflict with each other. French missionaries, often the first white men to explore new territory, worked continuously to convert the Indians to Christianity.

Most French and Spanish colonists were men—soldiers, traders, or clergy. They made use of native people to do the labor of farming, trapping, and mining as much as possible. The

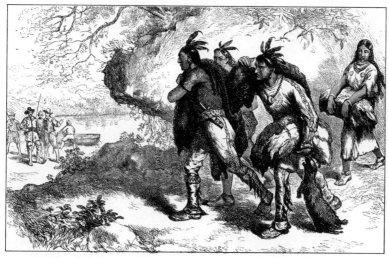

The Indians of North America willingly traded their rich furs for the white man's metal tools and firearms.

soldiers and traders often married Indian women so that people of mixed blood soon became an important element in the population of French and Spanish colonies. Europeans remained a minority in the colonial population.

The English took another approach. Trade, especially the fur trade, was important to them, but the land they claimed produced neither the quality nor the quantity of furs that came from the Canadian forests. What the British did find on their land was the sacred native tobacco plant. When tobacco was introduced to Europe, it was an instant success. The use of tobacco quickly passed from a fad to a habit among Europeans. Once the demand was created, the English decided to turn the American wilderness into a garden to satisfy it. Tobacco was to be supplied to trading

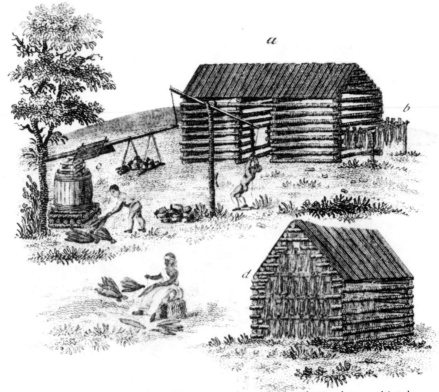

A tobacco plantation in colonial Virginia: a) common tobacco house; b) tobacco hanging on a scaffold; c) the operation of sizing tobacco; d) tobacco curing shed.

> # Twenty Dollars Reward.
>
> RAN away from the subscribers, living at New Rochelle, on Sunday evening, the 9th instant; two indented GERMAN SERVANTS: John Jacob Wittmer, belonging to Mr. Lispenard, about five feet five inches high, well set, has a remarkable large head, short neck and broad face; halts as he walks, his right leg being much shorter than the left; had on, or took with him when he went off, a blue broad cloth coat, with brass buttons, short white waistcoat, with red embroidered flowers; corduroy breeches; light coloured worsted stockings; new shoes, and new round hat, with a band and buckle. Mr. Williams's servant is a tall slim fellow, five feet eleven inches high; somewhat freckled; long hair, tyed behind; had on a mixed blue and white coat; black breeches; and took with him a pair of clouded overalls, red, blue and white, which he may probably wear. Whoever apprehends the above servants, and will bring them to their masters, at this place, shall receive the above reward, or ten dollars for either of them, with an allowance for all reasonable charges.
>
> LEONARD LISPENARD, jun.
> DANIEL WILLIAMS.
>
> New Rochelle, October 13, 1785.   33-6

A poster offering a reward for the return of indentured servants who have run away from their masters

companies by plantations that they established. Laborers were to be brought from home. Trading companies were "given" lands on which to start colonies. Rich men were given allotments of land for each immigrant they transported to the colonies. Poor men were promised land as an inducement to come as indentured servants.

The men and women who indentured themselves were generally the oppressed members of their society—people of the lowest classes who were, in addition, often paupers, debtors, and criminals. They "indentured" themselves as laborers for a specified time, from four to seven years. They were promised land at the end of their service. In the early years not many of the colonists outlived their period of indenture so that they could claim their land and freedom. One-third to one-half of the settlers who came to Virginia in the first 20 years of colonization died within a few months of their arrival. But the indentured laborers soon realized that they could slip into the wilderness and have all the land they wanted without working out their contracts.

The English also did their best to use Indian labor on the tobacco plantations. They enslaved Indians captured in war and sent them to plantations far from their homes. But the Indians were failures as slaves. They resisted the back-breaking plantation labor and they died like flies from the combined effects of strange climate, poor living conditions, and diseases. They regularly chose to kill themselves and their children rather than endure slavery. Thus the plantations faced a continual labor shortage; other laborers had to be found. In 1619 the first African slaves reached Virginia. By the time of the Revolution, there were 400,000 slaves in the colonies, three-fourths of them in the South.

In New England colonists were likely to be religious dissenters who were looking for a safe place to practice their unorthodox beliefs. Because this area was not suitable for large plantations, people settled closer together. Towns sprang up, and the townspeople, like those of the Old World, engaged in trade and manufacturing. Craftsmen and skilled laborers from the mother country used the raw materials of the region to manufacture goods that the colonists needed. The forests were shaped into "Yankee" ships. The ships brought molasses from the West Indies to New England, where it was made into rum. The rum was traded in Africa for black tribesmen who were transported to the American colonies as slaves. This "three-cornered" trade brought prosperity, more colonists, and greater independence.

Thus, by various methods, white men established themselves in North America, in colonies built on a foundation of economic ambition and territorial interest. The competition and hostility of the European states were transplanted in the new land. The French, English, Dutch, Spanish, and others schemed and struggled to secure their own colonies and to discourage all the others. When conflicts came, white men looked upon the native people as pawns in their strategies.

3. *Two Cultures Meet*

The story of the first Thanksgiving is one of America's favorites. The Plymouth settlers were not looking for trouble with the Indians. They had trouble enough with hunger, cold, disease, and fear. They were marooned in a wilderness half a world away from the palaces, cathedrals, cities, and armies of Europe. The members of the Plymouth colony would probably all have vanished, as the first English settlers on Roanoke Island did, if the Indians had not taken pity on them. The Indians brought them gifts of food and offered goodwill and friendship. The settlers survived, and the Indians taught them wilderness skills and maize culture. Then they left them in peace to tend their gardens.

Other white colonies along the eastern seaboard were also established with the help of the native people, but white men said their thanks to God, not to the Indians. Shipload after shipload of colonists and their goods poured into the coastal settlements. The Indians traded the riches of their country for the trinkets of civilization. The settlers' little gardens became fields, and fences divided the cultivated countryside from the wilderness. By the time the Indians realized that the white men planned to have everything, it was already too late to push them back into the sea.

Within 15 years of the Jamestown settlement, the Powhatans were fighting to put a stop to white expansion. In New England peace was maintained for over 50 years, but the exploitation and humiliation of the Indians by white colonists produced increasing tension. Among those affected by the tension were the Wampanoags, the people who had first befriended the Plymouth settlers. By 1675 their young chief Metacomet (named King Philip by whites) had decided that the only solution for his people was to drive the whites out of their land. Philip led a small alliance of New England tribes in attacks against the white settlements. He managed to keep up the hostilities for over a year.

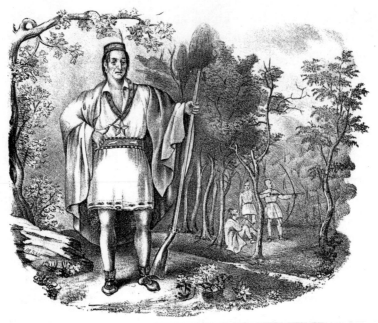

Metacomet, who was called King Philip by whites, led one of the earliest efforts to resist the white invasion of Indian lands.

The well-known raids on settlements up and down the Connecticut River, including the attack on Deerfield, Massachusetts, were part of what came to be called King Philip's War. But eventually Philip's allies began to desert him. He was betrayed, and he and his people were hunted down and killed. Such unsuccessful attempts to check the white invasion were only the first in a series of conflicts that continued for over 200 years.

Whenever two cultures meet, it is the rule that although both are changed, the less complex of the two changes most. The changes are not always voluntary, and they are not always for the good. In America, white men eagerly accepted the tobacco, maize, and furs the Indians brought them. Red men, in turn, were impressed by the products of European technology—metal tools and vessels, firearms, cotton cloth, bright, uniform glass beads.

They were anxious to acquire these things from the newcomers. But the trade that developed brought changes that resulted in the destruction of many Indian societies in colonial times.

The improved tools and guns made work a little easier and life a little better for the Indians. A temporary period of prosperity followed. But once Indians became accustomed to the trade goods, they became necessities rather than novelties and luxuries. If a man's enemies had firearms, it was essential to his survival that he also have a gun in working order and ammunition for it. Since Indians could not make these things, they were soon dependent on their trade with white men. When they fought as allies of white men against other Indians, they were usually protecting their own source of supplies from another tribe that had always been the enemy. Only a few were shrewd enough to see that, in the long run, most tribes really had more in common with their red enemies than they did with their white allies.

During the colonial era, the rapidly growing white population also affected the economic foundation of Indian life. Game and fur animals fled settled neighborhoods. When game became scarce, the Indians' need for white goods, including foodstuffs, increased. To supply these needs by means of trade, competition for the remaining animals was intensified. The process was hurried along by the business practices of the white traders who suspended fair play and honesty in the Indian trade without fear of consequences. The trader's object was to get rich quick. Thus white men paid for fortunes in furs with relatively inexpensive, everyday manufactured goods. This was possible because the Indians had no way of knowing the comparative value of the things they bought and sold, and, in most cases, they had no choice of markets. The monopoly that most white traders enjoyed was not advantage enough, however. They cheated in weighing, measuring, and counting. They sold watered rum, adulterated gun powder, and shoddy goods of all kinds. When the traders' dishonesty became too gross, the Indians did complain and some-times colonial administrators, anxious to avoid Indian trouble, would crack down on the worst abuses for a time. But the reforms never lasted long. The Indians also did away with some of the worst crooks themselves, but there were always others to take their places.

The more the Indians trapped and hunted to pay for the over-priced trade goods, the sooner they exhausted the animals that were their wealth. To make up for increasing shortages of pelts, Indians pushed out of their normal hunting grounds into the ter-ritory of other tribes. This competition brought continual warfare. Because survival was at stake, the conflicts became larger, more destructive, and more frequent than in precontact days. Some-times defeated tribes or villages were absorbed into the victorious tribe; sometimes they moved away into new territory. Those who went west found the white traders not far behind. Those who stayed near their old homes were bound to become poorer and poorer as their resources disappeared.

As white men crowded into unsettled areas, Indians were pressured to "sell" their lands. For a white man to own property, he needed a document showing that the previous owner had given up title to the land. Because white governments recog-nized Indian ownership of the land, they "treated with" tribal leaders to get them to sign such documents. They regarded the tribes as sovereign nations and the chiefs as kings who had the power to sign away tribal lands. Whites were not above using illegal or unethical means to get the signatures. Treaty discussions were always begun with large gifts of liquor for the Indians. It was much easier to defraud them when they were thoroughly befuddled. White men also did not hesitate to lie about the terms of the treaties or to conceal some of the conditions when they thought the Indians would object to them. They almost always made promises that they could not or would not keep.

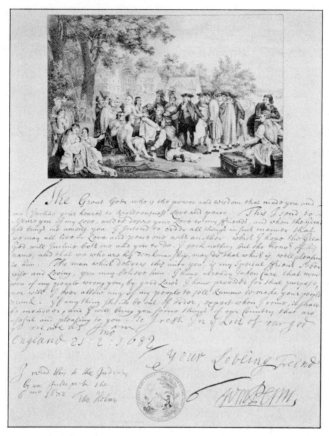

In 1682, William Penn signed a treaty with the Delaware Indians who lived in Pennsylvania. The treaty was honored for as long as Penn lived, but after his death it was ignored and the Delawares lost their land.

The terms of the treaties followed a formula. By signing the treaty, two free and independent peoples—the Indians and the whites—guaranteed their conduct in the future; there would be peace and friendship between them forever. The Indian nation agreed to give up its claim to the lands described in the treaty; the white government agreed to pay the monies and goods listed, usually in the form of yearly payments, or annuities. The whites guaranteed the Indians the right to enjoy their remaining land forever and the freedom to protect it from trespassers. Treaties of peace following a war were similar, but the lands described were claimed by "right of conquest."

Once they had title to the lands, the whites preferred that the Indians clear out altogether. Those who chose to stay near their old homes were reduced to poverty by the loss of their lands. The payments they received were always ridiculously small, even for those times. All too often the payments stopped before the full price was paid.

In the Northeast, Indians lived on the edges of white society in poverty and degradation. Men who had earned their place in society by hunting and fighting no longer had anything to do. As their needs increased, they were likely to go into debt or steal to provide for their families. Idle, poor, and without hope, some of them occupied themselves with drinking, fighting, and making mischief of other kinds. But guilty or innocent, all Indians were treated with mistrust and contempt by white settlers. Towns made special laws regulating the conduct of Indians, but Indians had no protection under white law. White men were not convicted of crimes against Indians, and Indians were not permitted to protect themselves against whites. In any quarrel with white men, an Indian was always wrong, even if he was defending his life and property. When white settlers broke the treaties by squatting on Indian lands, white governments protected the settlers, not Indian treaty rights.

Along with the cultural baggage that white men imported to the New World were the famous old plagues of Europe. Such contagious diseases as smallpox, measles, tuberculosis, typhoid, and cholera had been thinning European populations for centuries. White men had developed some resistance to them. Some were not infected even when they were exposed, and some managed to survive the diseases. (The familar pock-marked face of colonial times was a badge of that survival.) But the native people of America had no physiological defenses against these

92

diseases. Their traditional methods of treating disease were worse than useless against them. When an epidemic struck an Indian village or encampment, there was seldom anyone left to bury the dead. Some tribes were so reduced by disease that they were absorbed into larger groups, and their own cultures became virtually extinct.

Indians were also exposed to that other crushing plague of white civilization, alcohol. In precontact times alcoholic drinks were not made in that area that became the United States. When the races met, alcohol was as strange to Indians as tobacco was to Europeans. The cultural exchange took place and, as usual, the Indians lost the most. Indians always used tobacco moderately, in ceremonial ways. It was considered a precious, even a holy, plant. But the Indians' use of alcohol was uncontrolled and destructive from the very beginning. White men encouraged and took advantage of the use of alcohol by Indians. They always gave generous gifts of liquor before any trading or bargaining took place. And liquor was always one of the first things offered in trade in a new locality.

Indians were soon acquainted with the evils of drink. Indian elders and wise men advised their younger brothers to avoid the use of alcohol. Some communities prohibited alcohol altogether. But these controls had small success. As conditions of life worsened for Indians, alcoholism became an increasingly serious social problem.

Although such problems affected all Indians, a few of the larger and stronger tribes managed to retain some land throughout the colonial period. But most Indian societies were broken and scattered. Indians were excluded from white society. They felt dishonored and hopeless, and their behavior reflected their loss of status and self-respect, as well as their loss of livelihood. Poverty, disease, and alcohol took their toll, and Indian populations declined rapidly.

Religion was another element of white civilization that affected the lives of the Indians. Indians learned about white men's religion from their earliest contacts with them. Missionaries of every denomination devoted themselves to wiping out native religion in order to replace it with some variety of Christianity. They began by telling the Indians how worthless and corrupt all their beliefs and practices were. They tried to convince them that life after death, truth, love, and goodness all flowed from Christianity. Generally, the missionaries were unsatisfied with the results of their evangelizing. Indians observed firsthand the charity, love, and justice of their white Christian brothers. Many decided to reject the Christian message.

But Indians found various ways of adapting to Christianity. Some tribes took the Christian god and Christian symbols into

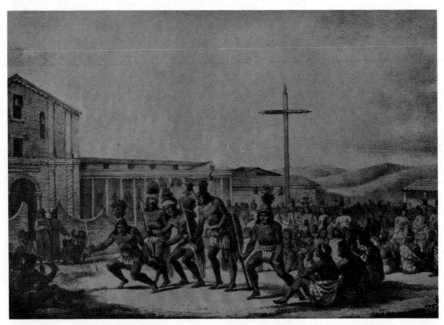

California Indians perform a native religious ritual following the Sunday service at a Christian mission. Such blendings of Christianity and native religions were common among American Indians.

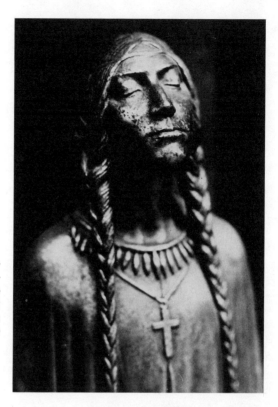

Kateri Tekawitha, a young Mohawk, was converted to Christianity in the 1670s. She became such a devout Christian that three centuries later she was a candidate for sainthood in the Catholic Church.

their own system of spirits and charms. They called on them as long as they seemed to help out in the hunt or with some other problem. Some Indians practiced both native and Christian religions side by side, living up to the missionaries' expectations in their presence and carrying on with their own religions in private. For some tribes the symbolism and rites of Christianity and native religions became so mixed that only an expert could tell where one left off and the other began. And some Indians did exactly what white missionaries wanted them to do—they became devout, committed, and loyal Christians. Christian Indians usually took their faith very seriously, which left them even more at the mercy of white men than their pagan brothers were.

From time to time, as the problems Indians faced grew more overwhelming, their need for inspiration and hope was filled by revivals of native religions, which usually had a strong addition of Christian concepts. The revival of Handsome Lake was such a movement. Handsome Lake (1735-1815) was a Seneca whose own life had been ruined by drinking. In 1799, during an illness, he had a great vision. As a result he set forth his "Good Message," a religious and moral code that combined old Iroquois and Quaker ideals. Included in the code was a prohibition against alcohol. Handsome Lake's "Good Message" was memorized and spread by disciples. Its object was to renew the moral and spiritual strength of his people.

Revivals such as Handsome Lake's give evidence of the influence that white religion had on the Indians of America. Indians found that white men were as eager to convert them to "civilization" as they were to convert them to Christianity. White men were convinced that they lived as men should live, even as God intended men to live. They were annoyed that Indians in their midst continued to act like Indians. They wanted them to stop moving around, to settle down and stay put. They wanted them to be farmers and to value property and possessions. White people put their faith in schools that were to teach these values to Indians.

The earliest schools for Indians were run by missionaries, like those established in 1568 by the Catholic clergy in Florida. They were primarily concerned with teaching Christianity, but very soon the curriculum was expanded to include the "arts of civilization"—reading, writing, rhetoric, literature, science. The goal of these white schools for Indians was to take the "Indianess" out of the Indians—to change their religion, values, and way of life.

By the time the Anglo-American colonies became the United States, the Indians had had 200 years of experience with white society. The problems Indians experienced in colonial times as a result of the contact with white men were not much different from those that exist today. It has often been suggested that the conflict was inevitable if "civilization" was to be advanced. A few men saw another way. America might have had a different history if the nation had followed the example of the Quakers in Pennsylvania, who lived in peace and brotherhood with the Indians for 75 years. Peaceful relations between Indians and whites existed in some other colonies as well. Roger Williams established his colony in Rhode Island and James Oglethorpe his in Georgia with the help of Indians. In these colonies Indians were treated with respect and honesty. Williams and Oglethorpe showed some gratitude and understanding toward the red men who shared their country with them, and the Indians repaid them

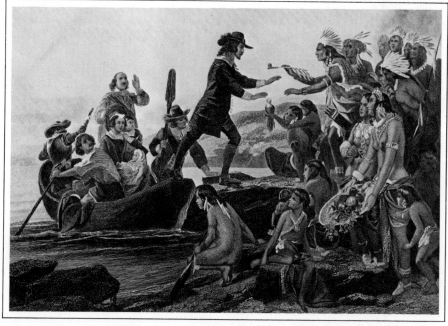

Roger Williams is greeted by friendly Indians on his arrival in Rhode Island. Indians were treated with respect and honesty in the colony that Williams established.

with trust and loyal friendship. But as more people crowded in, Pennsylvania, Rhode Island, and Georgia went the way of their neighbors, and their example faded from memory.

4. *The Colonial Balance of Power*

Indians were involved in the wars for domination of North America for decades. They fought with white allies, and their fortunes rose and fell with the success or failure of those allies. In the 18th century the competition between the French and British for the fur trade grew into full scale war in the Northeast. The Iroquois, allies of the British, were a powerful factor in the final defeat of the French. After the fall of Quebec in 1759, France was no longer a power in America.

The Indians who had been allies of the French feared further white expansion west of the Alleghenies. Therefore, a number of tribes united under the Ottawa chief Pontiac to resist the British

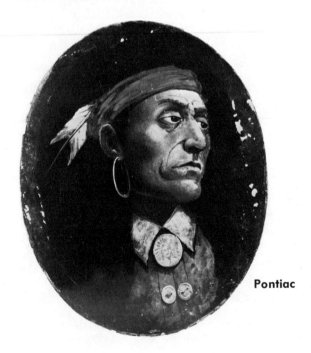

Pontiac

in the Great Lakes area. The war with Pontiac worried the British. They preferred to trade with the Indians rather than fight with them. Moreover, the British were no more in favor of white expansion in the area than the Indians were; it was already clear to them that white settlement ruined the fur trade. Thus in 1763, the year the treaty of peace was signed with France, the British forbade any further settlement west of the Appalachians and ordered white men already in the area to get out. The British made other attempts to come to terms with the Indians by settling the boundaries of Indian lands permanently. By means of this settlement, the Iroquois in the Northeast and the Creeks and Cherokees in the Southeast retained a large share of their original land.

The Iroquois, Creeks, and Cherokees held a secure position as allies of the British, but this position became a liability when the American colonies won freedom from British rule. American settlements had often suffered from Indian attacks directed by the British during the Revolution. The war left most Americans, especially those on the frontiers, with a seething hatred of both the British and their Indian allies. That hatred was easily stretched to cover all Indians, whether they took part in the hostilities or not.

Before the Revolution each group of colonists had been held in check, to some degree, by the colonies of other great powers nearby. Some Indian tribes were able to fit into this balance of power. They received consideration from colonies that needed their military assistance. After the war, the new nation took control of the territory previously held by the colonial powers. But the situation was changed, for now all white men were *Americans*, united in their identity and in their ambitions. America was nation-building. To stay independent of European domination and to take its place as a world power, the new American government pursued wealth, territory, and power. No prophet was needed to predict what lay ahead for the American natives.

TRIBES AND LANGUAGE FAMILIES

Scholars have made many attempts to classify Indian languages into related families, but they have not yet devised a system of classification that is entirely successful. The following list of major Indian tribes grouped in language families is based on a classification system that is familiar and widely accepted.

Athabaskan

Beaver
Carrier
Chipewyan
Haida
Hare
Hupa
Kutchin
Navajo
Sarsi
Sekani
Slave
Tlingit

Algonquian

Abnaki
Algonquin
Arapaho
Blackfoot
Blood
Cheyenne
Conestoga
Cree
Delaware
Fox
Gros Ventres
Kickapoo
Massachusetts
Menomini
Miami
Micmac
Mohegan
Ojibwa (Chippewa)
Ottawa

Penobscot
Peoria
Pequot
Piegan
Potawatomi
Powhatan
Sauk
Shawnee
Susquehanna
Wampanoag
Yurok

Iroquoian

Cayuga
Cherokee
Erie
Huron
Iroquois
Mohawk
Oneida
Onondaga
Seneca
Tuscarora

Siouan

Assiniboin
Chiwere
Crow
Dakota (Sioux)
Hidatsa
Iowa
Kansa
Mandan

Minitari
Missouri
Omaha
Osage
Oto
Ponca
Winnebago

Muskogean

Calusa
Chickasaw
Choctaw
Creek
Natchez
Seminole
Timacua

Caddoan

Arikara
Caddo
Pawnee
Wichita

Sahaptin

Cayuse
Nez Perce
Wallawalla
Yakima

Penutian

Chinook
Maidu
Tsimshian

Uto-Aztecan

Comanche
Hopi
Kiowa
Paiute
Papago
Pima
Ute

Mosanic

Coeur d'Alene
Colville
Flathead
Kalispel
Kwakiutl
Nootka
Salish

Hokan

Havasupai
Karankawa
Mojave
Pomo
Tonkawa
Walapai
Yavapai
Yuma

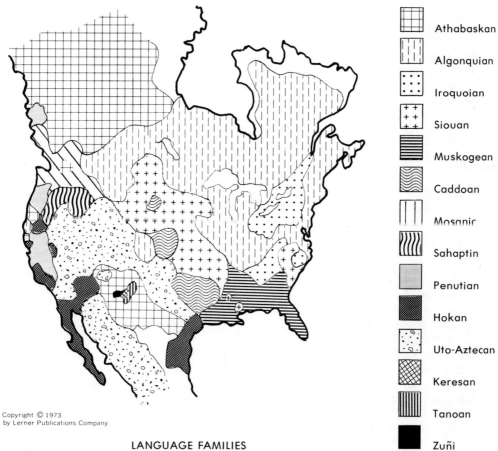

Athabaskan
Algonquian
Iroquoian
Siouan
Muskogean
Caddoan
Mosanic
Sahaptin
Penutian
Hokan
Uto-Aztecan
Keresan
Tanoan
Zuñi

LANGUAGE FAMILIES

... INDEX ...

pemmican, 73
Pennacook, 61
Pennsylvania, treatment of Indians in, 97-98
Penobscot, 61
Peoria, 61
Pequot, 61
Pima, 56
Plateau, The, 49, 51, 52-54
Plymouth colony, 87
Ponca, 70
Ponce de Leon, 80
Pontiac, 98-99
population, Indian, 38-39
Potawatomi, 61
potlach, 48
pottery, 18, 21, 58
Powhatan, 64, 65-66
Pueblo Indians, 55-58, 72
pueblos, 55-58

Quakers, 97

Raleigh, Sir Walter, 80
religion, Indian, 32-36, 56-57; compared to European religion, 77
Revolution, American, 99
Rhode Island, treatment of Indians in, 97-98

sachem, 64
Salish, 47
salmon, 46, 52
Sarsi, 45
Sauk and Fox, 61
Sekani, 45
Seneca, 61, 64
shaman, 35
Shawnee, 64
Shoshone, 53, 54, 70
Siouan language, 61, 70
Sioux (Dakota), 61, 71
Slave, 45
social organization, Indian, 25-32, 65-66

society, definition of, 9
Southwest, 50, 51, 55-60, 73
Spain, colonization by, 80, 81-82, 83-84
Spokane, 52
Susquehanna, 61
sweating, 22-23, 36

Tanoan language, 56
Timacua, 65
tipi, 73
Tlingit, 47
tobacco: as English plantation crop, 84-86; used by Indians, 21, 36, 93
totem, 26-27
totem pole, 8, 48
treaties, 90-92
tribe, 29
Tsimshian, 47
tumpline, 22
Tunica, 64
Tuscarora, 64

Ute, 70
Uto-Aztecan language, 53, 56

voyageurs, 83

Walapai, 56
Wallawalla, 52
Wampanoag, 61, 87
warfare: among Plains Indians, 75; among Woodland Indians, 66-68
weaving, 59
wigwam, 62
Williams, Roger, 97-98
Winnebago, 61
Wisconsin Glacier, 11, 13
witchcraft, 32, 35
woodcarving, 48-49
writing, systems of, 8, 9

Yakima, 52
Yavapai, 56
Yuma, 56

Zuñi, 56